Strategies Techniques and Approaches to Thinking

Case Studies in Clinical Nursing

Sandra Luz Martinez de Castillo, EdD, RN
Instructor, Department of Nursing
Contra Costa College
San Pablo, California

W.B. SAUNDERS COMPANY
A Division of Harcourt Brace & Company
Philadelphia London Toronto Sydney

W.B. SAUNDERS COMPANY
A Division of Harcourt Brace & Company
Independence Square West
Philadelphia, PA 19106

STRATEGIES, TECHNIQUES, AND APPROACHES TO THINKING:
Case Studies in Clinical Nursing ISBN 0–7216–7648–0

Printed in the United States of America.

Last digit is the print number: 9 8 7 6 5 4 3 2 1

Dedication

Para mi mamá, Blanca Rosa Martínez, que me dio la visión.
Para mi papá, Miguel Duarte Martínez, que me dio la opportunidad.
Para mis hijos, Mike, Marisa, Raquel, Isaac, que me dieron su apoyo.
Para mi nieta, Rebeca BlancaLuz, que me dio su risa.
Especialmente para Dios – por todo.

ACKNOWLEDGMENTS

I am grateful for all the feedback and support given to me during the preparation of this book. I would like to extend my appreciation to Lynda Schweid, Maryanne Werner-McCullough, Sharon Reder, Al Lamons, Barbara Santina, Mary Anne Anderson, Cheri Etheredge, Roberta Hoffman, Saul Jones, Maureen Garretson, and Vickie Jeung, the nursing faculty at Contra Costa College, for their willingness to listen and support this book. I would also like to acknowledge Sharon Johnson, nursing instructor at Los Medanos College, for supporting and using parts of this book with her students.

I am especially grateful to Margaret Sutter, RN, CDE, Lynne Booth, RN, ONC, and Judy Kohn, RN, BSN, CDE, John Muir Medical Center, for their willingness to share their knowledge and expertise in the development of numerous scenarios.

I would like to especially acknowledge Maryanne Werner-McCullough, my dear friend and colleague, for listening, reviewing, editing, and making suggestions during the past year.

To my family, Rosie, Panch, Mike, for their words of encouragement and support and to my special friend, Shirley Archuleta, for her words of wisdom.

Finally, to Yolanda Baldovinos and Fred Lopez for their genuine friendship and love. Thanks for making my life easier.

Reviewer Listing

Rebecca Lynn Agnew, MSN, RN
Mercy School of Nursing
Pittsburgh, Pennsylvania

Michele A. Gerwick, MSN, RN
Doctoral Candidate
Indiana University of Pennsylvania
Indiana, Pennsylvania

Mary Taylor Martof, EdD, RN
Louisiana State University Medical Center
School of Nursing
New Orleans, Louisiana

Carol A. Melin, MN, RN
South Dakota State University
Brookings, South Dakota

Patricia L. Newland, RN, MS
Broome Community College
Binghamton, New York

C. Sue Snyder, PhD, RN, C
Associate Professor
Department of Nursing and Allied Health Professions
Indiana University of Pennsylvania
Indiana, Pennsylvania

Preface

Dear Nursing Student:

You have chosen a wonderful profession! During the next few months, you will be learning many nursing concepts, principles, and skills and will have the opportunity to apply the nursing skills in the clinical environment. You will also meet many nurses who, through their clinical experience and knowledge, utilize critical thinking skills to make patient care decisions.

This manual is designed to assist you to develop critical thinking skills. The manual is divided into four sections to coincide with your learning needs. It is very important to have a strong theoretical foundation; therefore, **Section One** is devoted to reinforcing concepts and principles pertinent to nursing practice. Knowledge is fundamental to using critical thinking skills, so take your time and work through the case studies and the learning activities. Every effort was made to develop short clinical case studies and patient care situations that are encountered in the clinical setting. The case studies in Section One have a dual purpose: (1) to reinforce fundamental concepts and principles and (2) to demonstrate how learned knowledge is applied in patient care situations.

Section Two is devoted to helping you prioritize and make sound clinical decisions. Similar to Section One, the case studies designed for this section focus on common clinical situations. You are encouraged to discuss and compare your decisions and rationales with your peers and your instructor. The process of *discussion* is very important to your learning. It is through the mutual sharing of knowledge, ideas, and experiences that you will learn how to prioritize and make clinical decisions based on sound rationales. The nursing process is included in this section to assist you in applying the components of assessment, nursing diagnosis, planning, and implementation.

Section Three presents clinical situations using an intershift report format. The presenting situation is given through the intershift report. Relevant and irrelevant information is provided in order to assist you to *analyze* and *interpret* data based on the presenting situation. Flow charts in the form of the patient's Nursing Care Rand/Kardex, Medication Record, Intake and Output Record, Nursing Notes, or History and Physical are provided to assist you in gathering further data. The twofold purpose of this activity is to help you (1) focus on gathering the data, both from the report and the flow charts, and (2) make relevant connections between the data.

Section Four presents answers for selected case studies. Case studies with answers are indicated by an asterisk following the title on the table of contents. Answers for other case studies are not provided so that students and instructors can have the opportunity for a more open dialogue during clinical conferences or class discussions.

Finally, the Critical Thinking Model provides a simple, yet logical, format for looking at the case studies. The Critical Thinking Model can be utilized in any clinical setting to assist you in the process of developing and utilizing critical thinking skills. I hope you will enjoy working with these activities and, most of all, that you enjoy the learning process!

The Publisher and I would appreciate any feedback you would be willing to provide on the classroom use of this text and its accompanying Instructor's Manual. We encourage you to contact the Publisher's web site at **www.wbsaunders.com** to share your comments and suggestions regarding these publications.

CONTENTS

SECTION ONE — COGNITIVE-BUILDING CRITICAL THINKING ACTIVITIES

SECTION TWO — PRIORITY-SETTING AND DECISION-MAKING ACTIVITIES

SECTION THREE — APPLYING THE CRITICAL THINKING MODEL

Notice

Nursing is an ever-changing field. Standard safety precautions must be followed, but as new research and clinical experience broaden our knowledge, changes in treatment and drug therapy become necessary or appropriate. Readers are advised to check the product information currently provided by the manufacturer of each drug to be administered to verify the recommended dose, the method and duration of administration, and contraindications. It is the responsibility of the treating physician, relying on experience and knowledge of the patient, to determine dosages and the best treatment of the patient. Neither the Publisher nor the editor assumes any responsibility for any injury and/or damage to persons or property.

The Publisher

SECTION ONE

Cognitive-Building Critical Thinking Activities

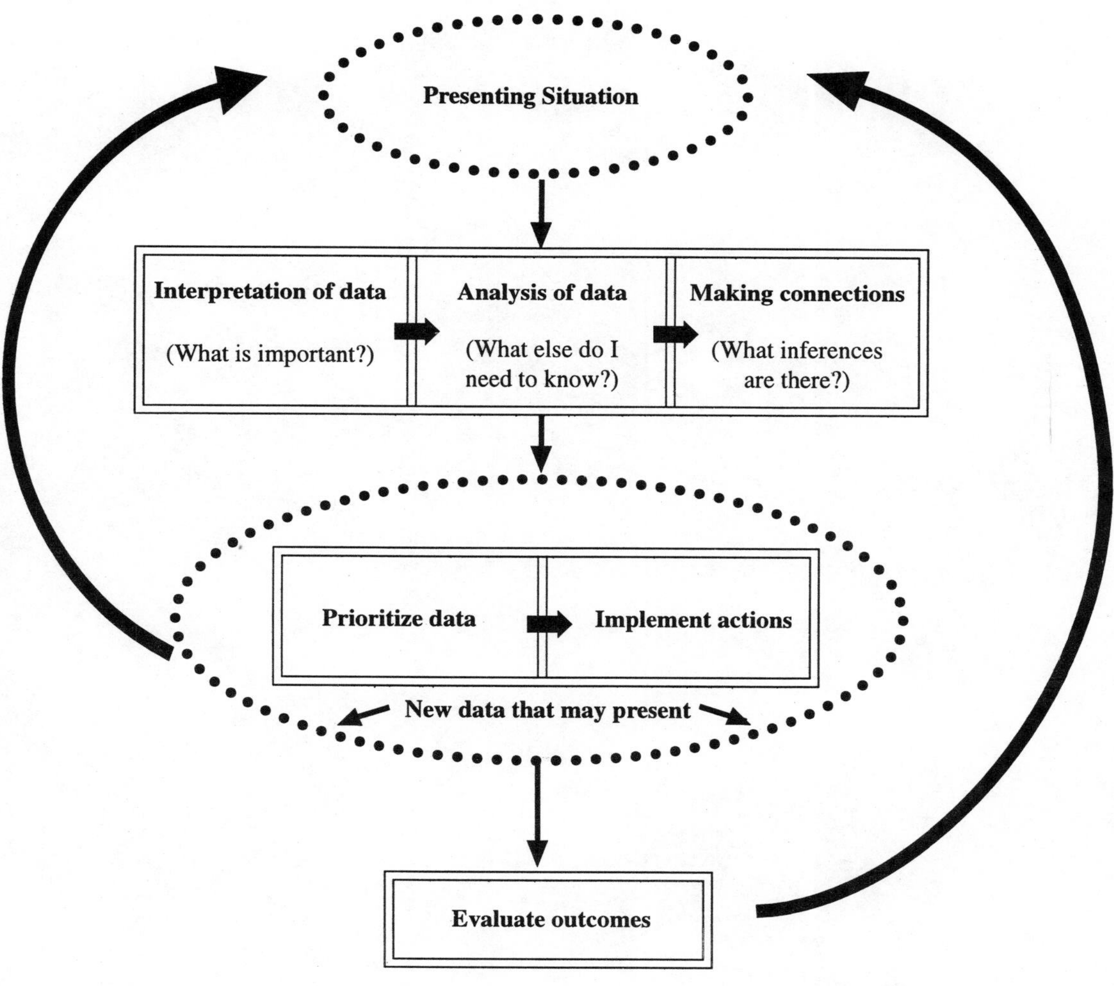

VITAL SIGNS

List the routes for taking a **temperature**:

1. ____________________
2. ____________________
3. ____________________
4. ____________________

Use the diagram to identify the **pulse sites** in the body.

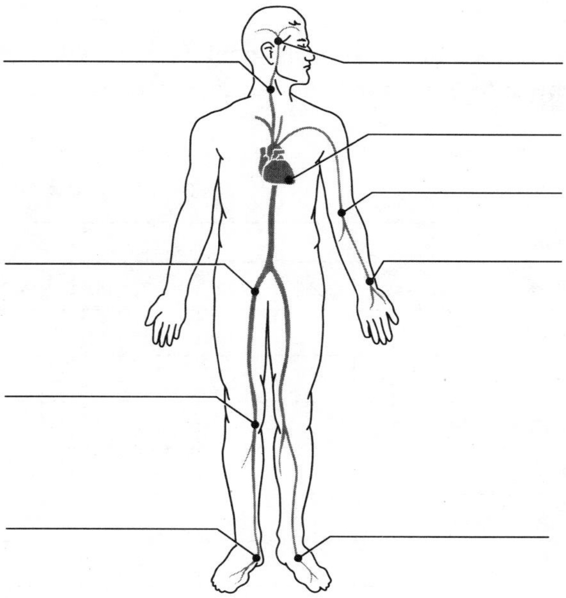

The **blood pressure** may be auscultated in the __________ & ____________ space.

Case Study: Stanley Moore has been having a high fever for 2 days. After visiting the physician's office, he was found to be febrile. Additionally, Mr. Moore is complaining of chills, night sweats, anorexia, and fatigue. He is admitted to the hospital. The physician's orders include vital signs every four hours. On admission he was experiencing pyrexia. His admission vital signs are T. 102.4° F. P. 96 - R. 26 BP 148/88.

Pertinent Terminology	Definition
Vital signs	
Temperature	
Pulse	
Respiration	
Blood Pressure	
Febrile	
Pyrexia	
Anorexia	
Fatigue	

From the case study, record today's date and the 0800 admission vital signs (VS) on the **Graphic Sheet** in the appropriate column. Enter the following vital signs for today:

1200 T. 103.6 - P. 108 - R. 32 BP 160/76

1600 T. 101.2 - P. 98 - R. 28 BP 154/82

2000 T. 100.0 - P. 80 - R. 24 BP 150/90

Record the 0800 VS for the next day: T. 99.6 - P. 72 - R. 18 BP 146/94
Draw a line between the temperature recordings to create a graph.

GRAPHIC SHEET

Date												
Time	0400	0800	1200	1600	2000	2400	0400	0800	1200	1600	2000	2400
40.0 C 104F												
39.4 103												
38.9 102												
38.3 101												
37.8 100												
37.2 99												
36.7 98												
36.1 97												
35.6 96												
Pulse		96	108	98	80			72				
Resp.		26	32	28	24			18				
B/P		148/88	160/76	154/82	150/90			146/94				

Interactive Activity: With a partner, identify the **normal range(s)** for the vital signs in the adult.

Body temperature **Oral** ____________________

Axillary ____________________

Rectal ____________________

Pulse _____________________________

Respirations _____________________________

Blood Pressure _____________________________

TEMPERATURE

The **body temperature** is regulated through the ________________________.

Body temperature remains constant through **heat production** and **heat loss**.

Factors that influence heat production:

- ☼ ____________________
- ☼ ____________________

Factors that influence heat loss:

- « ____________________
- « ____________________
- « ____________________
- « ____________________

Body temperature is affected by:

1. ____________________
2. ____________________
3. ____________________
4. ____________________
5. ____________________
6. ____________________

Case Study: Mrs. Ray, 79 yrs. old, was brought to the Emergency Department after having been found unconscious in her home. The physician has admitted her with the diagnosis of heatstroke. On admission the vital signs are: T. 40.5° C. - P. 100 - R. 16, BP 118/64. Her skin is flushed and feels hot and dry. She is complaining of nausea. The physician orders the temperature to be monitored every hour.

Pertinent Terminology	Definition
Temperature	________________________
Hyperthermia	________________________
Hypothermia	________________________
Heatstroke	________________________
Conduction	________________________
Convection	________________________
Evaporation	________________________
Radiation	________________________

From the case study, explain how the **evaporation factor** contributed to Mrs. Ray's development of heatstroke:

____

☞ **Fill in the thermometers** to reflect the temperature readings (both Celsius and Fahrenheit) for your shift on Mrs. Ray:

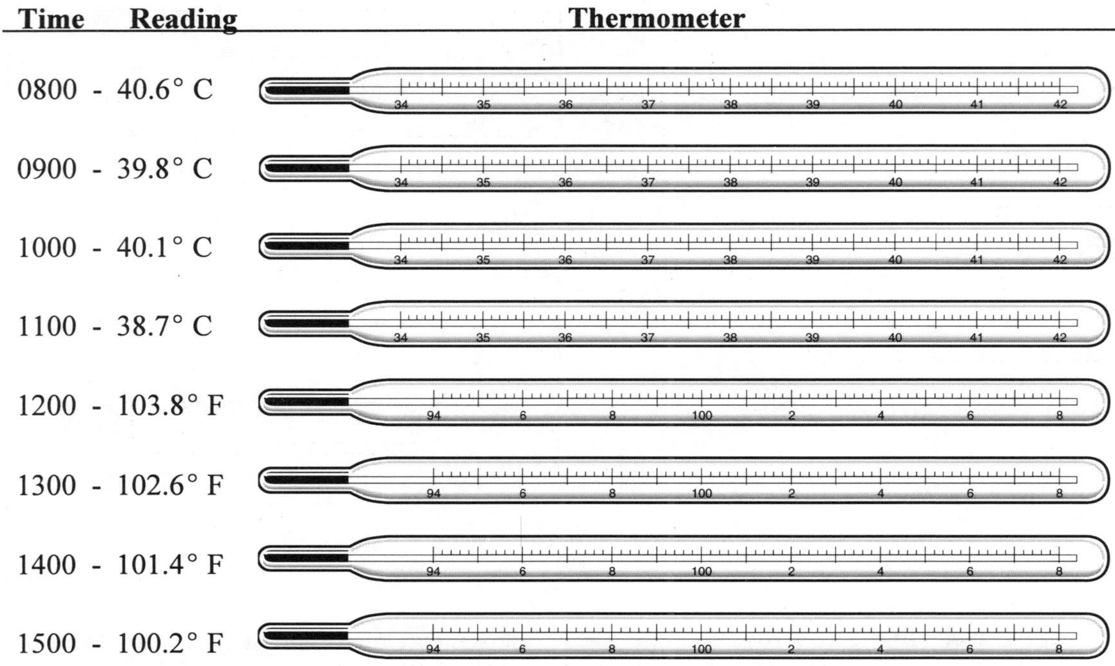

Interactive Activity: Graph the temperature readings for your shift. Draw a line between each temperature recording. Compare the **Temperature Recording Sheet** with a partner.

TEMPERATURE RECORDING SHEET

	Time	0800	0900	1000	1100	1200	1300	1400	1500
40.6C	105F								
40.0	104								
39.4	103								
38.9	102								
38.3	101								
37.8	100								
36.7	98								
36.1	97								
35.6	96								

PULSE

The normal **pulse rate range** for an adult is: ______________________________.

The **pulse characteristics** includes a description of the _________, _________, and ____________________ of the pulse.

The **pulse rate** is affected by:

1. ______________________
2. ______________________
3. ______________________
4. ______________________
5. ______________________
6. ______________________
7. ______________________
8. ______________________

Draw circles on the diagram that identify the sites where the **pulse** is found in the body.

Case Study: Mr. Sanchez, 52 yrs. old, has been complaining of a rapid heart beat. He says that it feels as if his "heart is racing." His wife took him to the Urgent Care Clinic where he was found to have an irregular pulse of 160 beats per minute (bpm) and was transferred to the hospital. On admission to the hospital his vital signs are T. 98.4 - P. 168 - R. 28, and BP 146/90. His skin is moist and he is very anxious. The physician orders the administration of cardiac medications and for the pulse to be monitored every two hours.

Pertinent Terminology	Definition
Pulse	
Stroke volume	
Cardiac output	
Pulse rhythm	
Pulse quality	
Tachycardia	
Bradycardia	
Arrhythmia	
Pulse deficit	

From the case study, use the admission pulse of 168 bpm to assist in identifying the words in the parenthesis that would **best describe** the characteristics of this pulse:

Pulse Characteristic	Descriptive Words	Selected Word(s)
Rate	(rapid, tachycardia, bradycardia, increased)	____________
Rhythm	(regular, irregular, abnormal, dysrhythmia)	____________
Quality	(weak, thready, bounding, difficult to palpate)	____________

Interactive Activity: With a partner, identify the **pulse site** in each diagram and **write in the reason** for checking the pulse from this area.

Pulse: ____________

Reason: ____________

Pulse: ____________

Reason: ____________

Pulse: ____________

Reason: ____________

Pulse: ____________

Reason: ____________

♡ The **apical pulse** is taken when ____________

To take an **apical pulse,** the stethoscope is placed on ____________

RESPIRATION

The normal **respiration rate range** for an adult is_______________________________.

The **characteristics of respiration** include a description of the __________, __________, and ________________ of the respirations.

The factors that affect the **characteristics of the respiration** include:

1.____________________________
2.____________________________
3.____________________________
4.____________________________
5.____________________________
6.____________________________
7.____________________________
8.____________________________
9.____________________________

A **normal** respiratory pattern consists of a full inspiration and a full expiration counted over one minute as the diagram illustrates:

One minute

Exp.

Insp.

The diagram demonstrates a _______________ respiratory pattern.

One minute

Exp.

Insp.

The diagram demonstrates a _______________

Case Study: Mr. Lee Kay has been a smoker for 20 years. He has noticed increased shortness of breath (SOB) for the past six months and is complaining of a productive cough with thick whitish phelgm. The nurse notices that his respiratory rate is 32, regular, and describes his lung sounds as fine crackling sounds heard on inspiration.

Pertinent Terminology	Definition
Respiration	
Tachypnea	
Bradypnea	
Eupnea	
Apnea	
Orthopnea	
Dyspnea	
Cheyne-Stokes	
Kussmaul	
Phlegm	

From the case study, use the respiratory rate of 32 to assist in identifying the words in the parenthesis that would **best describe** the characteristics of this breathing pattern:

Respiratory Characteristic	Descriptive Words	Selected Word(s)
Rate	(eupnea, tachypnea, bradypnea, apnea)	____________
Depth	(deep, full inspiration/expiration, short, shallow)	____________
Rhythm	(regular, irregular)	____________

✎✎ **Draw a line** to match the **identified lung sounds** below with the appropriate description:

Wheeze	crackling sound, may be fine or coarse, heard frequently on inspiration.
Crackle	coarse, harsh, loud sound, best heard on expiration
Gurgle	continuous high pitched muscial sound best heard on expiration

✎✎ **Circle** the lung sound that best describes Mr. Kay's lung sounds.

Interactive Activity: Draw a diagram that respresents each of the respiratory patterns identified in each box. Compare and discuss your diagrams with a partner.

1 minute

Respiration Pattern: Apnea

1 minute

Respiration Pattern: Tachypnea

1 minute

Respiration Pattern: Cheyne-Stokes

1 minute

Respiration Pattern: Kussmaul

BLOOD PRESSURE

The average **blood pressure** for an adult is ______________________.

Factors that affect the **blood pressure** include:

1. ______________________
2. ______________________
3. ______________________
4. ______________________
5. ______________________
6. ______________________
7. ______________________
8. ______________________
9. ______________________
10. ______________________

Identify the parts of the following items used in obtaining a blood pressure:

Case Study: Mr. Harold is a 65-yr.-old African-American man. He goes weekly to the Hypertension Clinic for blood pressure checks. He has a 20-year history of smoking 2 packs of cigarettes a day. His father died from heart disease and his brother also has hypertension. His current blood pressure (BP) reading is 174/104 and he is complaining of a headache and dizziness when getting up in the morning.

Pertinent Terminology	Definition
Blood pressure	
Systolic pressure	
Diastolic pressure	
Korotkoff's sounds	
Pulse pressure	
Hypertension	
Hypotension	
Orthostatic hypotension	
Auscultatory gap	

From the case study, identify the **factors** that predisposed Mr. Harold for developing hypertension:

______________________ ______________________ ______________________

______________________ ______________________ ______________________

§ The clinic nurse monitors Mr. Harold's blood pressure for three days:

Day I	
11:00 AM	210/110
11:15 AM	202/104
11:30 AM	190/98

Day 2	
11:00 AM	188/100
11:15 AM	170/98
11:30 AM	164/94

Day 3	**11:00 AM**
Lying	178/100
Sitting	166/90
Standing	150/90

Interactive Activity: Record the blood pressure readings on the flow sheet using the symbol "V" to identify the systolic reading and the symbol "Λ" for the diastolic reading. Connect both symbols with a straight line. Identify the orthostatic blood pressure readings with the appropriate symbols. Compare your flow sheet with a partner.

BLOOD PRESSURE FLOW SHEET

Date	Day 1			Day 2			Day 3			
Time	11:00	11:15	11:30	11:00	11:15	11:30	11:00			
240										
230										
220										
210										
200										
190										
180										
170										
160										
150										
140										
130										
120										
110										
100										
90										
80										
70										
60										

BODY MECHANICS

List the factors that affect a patient's ability to move and maintain body alignment:

1.______________________________
2.______________________________
3.______________________________
4.______________________________
5.______________________________
6.______________________________

Use the diagram to identify the **four basic principles** of body mechanics:

1.____________________________
2.____________________________
3.____________________________
4.____________________________

Case Study: Mrs. Wiley has suffered a cerebral vascular accident (CVA) and as a result has left-sided hemiplegia. The M.D. orders for Mrs. Wiley to be out of bed (OOB) twice a day and to be turned every two hours while in bed. The RN asks the staff to do passive range of motion (ROM) exercises to her left side and to use supportive devices to ensure proper body alignment. Mrs. Wiley is to do active ROM with her right side.

Pertinent Terminology	Definition
Range of motion	
Active ROM	
Passive ROM	
CVA	
Hemiplegia	
Alignment	
Hand roll	
Trochanter roll	
Footboard	
Plantar flexion	
Flaccid	

From the case study, **(1) identify** the **major body areas** that would require special nursing care, **(2) select** the most appropriate **supportive device** from the list that will assist in maintaining proper body alignment for Mrs. Wiley, and **(3) state the complication** the nursing care will prevent:

Hand roll	Trochanter roll	Pillow	Trapeze bar	Sandbag	Footboard

Major Body Area	Supportive Device	This helps to prevent

Select the Activities of Daily Living (ADLs) below that Mrs. Wiley can perform **independently** throughout the day which encourage **active ROM** to the **right side** of her body:

- ☐ Brushing her teeth
- ☐ Transferring OOB
- ☐ Flexing/extending ankle
- ☐ Combing her hair
- ☐ Ambulating
- ☐ Standing
- ☐ Washing face
- ☐ Feeding herself

Interactive Activity: With a partner, beginning with number 1, **number the following interventions** in the order necessary to assist Mrs. Wiley to transfer from the bed to a wheelchair:

_____ Place wheelchair at a 45° angle to the bed

_____ Lock the wheelchair brakes

_____ Assist Mrs. Wiley to a sitting position at the side of the bed

_____ Provide instructions to Mrs. Wiley

_____ Cross Left lower extremity over Right lower extremity

_____ Have Mrs. Wiley pivot toward the wheelchair

_____ Lower Mrs. Wiley into the wheelchair

_____ Stand Mrs. Wiley, support Left lower extremity

_____ Have Mrs. Wiley support Left upper extremity with Right upper extremity

HYGIENE

The **purpose of providing a bath** is to:

1. ____________________________
2. ____________________________
3. ____________________________
4. ____________________________
5. ____________________________

Identify the various methods of bathing:

1. ____________________________
2. ____________________________
3. ____________________________
4. ____________________________

Place a "✓" mark on the information that best describes the following.

Early Morning care includes:

- ☐ Starting the bath early in the morning.
- ☐ Providing/assisting with oral hygiene.
- ☐ Washing face and hands.
- ☐ Offering bedpan, urinal or assisting to the bathroom.

Hour of Sleep (HS) care includes:

- ☐ Providing a back rub for the patient.
- ☐ Straightening the bed linens.
- ☐ Providing/assisting with oral hygiene.
- ☐ Take the vital signs.

Case Study: Mrs. Hailey, 88 yrs. old, has been in the hospital for two days with an irregular heartbeat. She is confused and just lies in bed. The RN informs you that Mrs. Hailey has urinary and bowel incontinence and is wearing an adult incontinence pad. Her skin is very fragile, she has several ecchymotic areas on the lower extremities, and she is wearing antiembolic stockings. Her toenails are long, yellowish, and thick. She has dried feces under her fingernails.

Pertinent Terminology	Definition
Antiembolic stockings	
Stomatitis	
Canthus	
Ecchymosis	
Perineum	
Labia majora	
Labia minora	
Prepuce	

Use the case study to identify the **most appropriate** nursing interventions for taking care of Mrs. Haileys's hands and feet. **Circle** the nursing interventions below that you would implement:

Nursing Interventions:

HANDS

1 Do nothing until the RN informs you.
2 Soak the hands for 10 minutes in lukewarm water.
3 Give the bath as usual, but do not soak the hands.
4 Use a green stick or Q-tip to remove the feces.
5 Cut the fingernails carefully to prevent further collection.

FEET

1 Remove the antiembolic stockings during the bath.
2 Soak the feet for 10 minutes in luke warm water.
3 Give a partial bath, apply lotion.
4 Dry well between the toes.
5 Cut the toenails carefully straight across.

✎ **Describe** the proper method for performing perineal care on a:

Female____

____

Male____

____

Interactive Activity: With a partner, identify the type of bath **most appropriate** for the following case scenarios:

Case Scenarios	Type of bath		
A 39-yr.-old female who had abdominal surgery and will be discharged this morning.	**Complete**	**Partial**	**Shower** (M.D. order/policy)
A 56-yr.-old patient admitted with lung problems and gets very short of breath with mild exertion.	**Complete**	**Partial**	**Shower**
A 23-yr.-old woman who is alert, but had a grand mal seizure two days ago.	**Complete**	**Partial**	**Shower**
A 46-yr.-old who had a motor vehicle accident (MVA) yesterday, suffered a mild concussion but no fractures.	**Complete**	**Partial**	**Shower**

INFECTION CONTROL/TRANSMISSION OF ORGANISMS

Provide examples of the following elements found in the **Chain of Infection**:

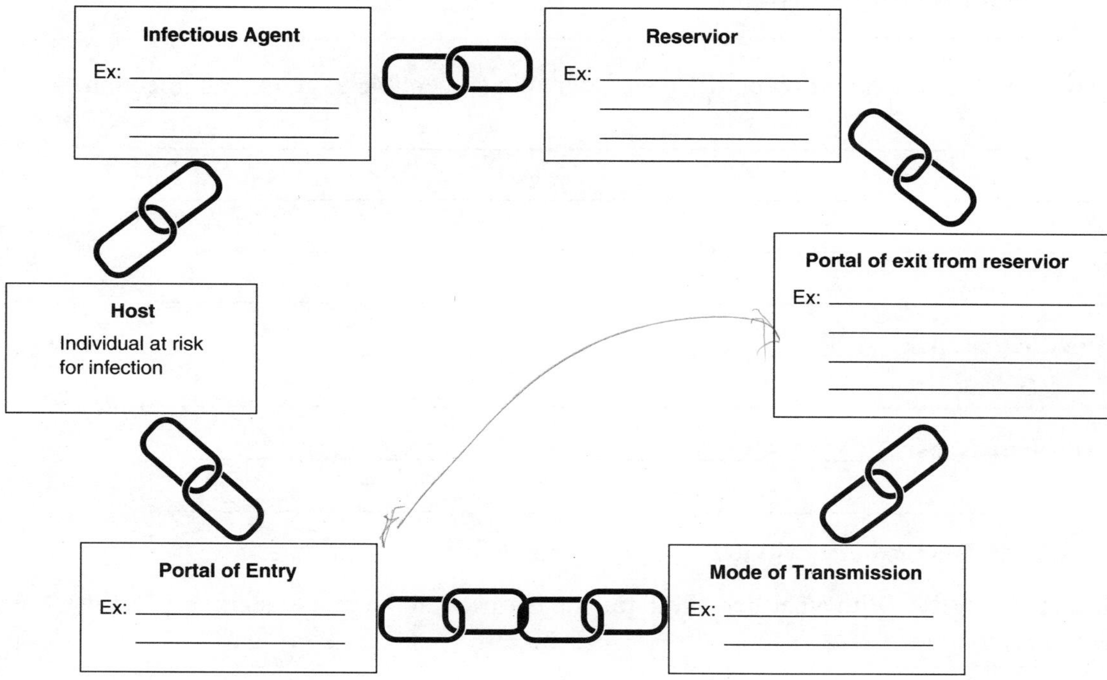

Case Study: Keli has recently begun nursing school. During her second week in the clinical setting, Keli takes care of Mr. Wu, a 79-yr.-old patient, who was admitted with dehydration. He has a recent history of shingles that is in the convalescent stage of illness. Mr. Wu's skin is very dry, his oral temperature is 100.4°F. His urine is very dark amber and his WBC is 13,000/mm^3.

Pertinent Terminology	Definition
Shingles	
Dehydration	
Incubation stage	
Prodromal stage	
Illness stage	
Convalescent stage	
Asepsis	
Nosocomial	

From the case study, identify the **factors** that make Mr. Wu susceptible for getting an infection?

______________________ ______________________

______________________ ______________________

Explain **why** each of the **factors** identified make Mr. Wu susceptible to getting an infection.

____

____

____

____

Define **medical asepsis**:____

____

Define **surgical asepsis**:____

____

In caring for Mr. Wu the nurse will use __________ asepsis.

Interactive Activity: With a partner, fill in the **diagrams** with the proper **elements in the Chain of Infection** as it applies to each situation:

1. A family member who has a cold stops in to visit Mr. Wu.

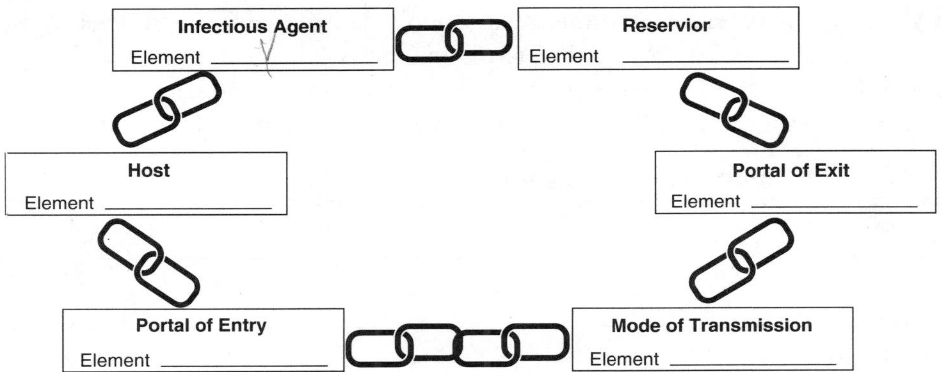

2. A nursing assistant goes from patient to patient without changing gloves.

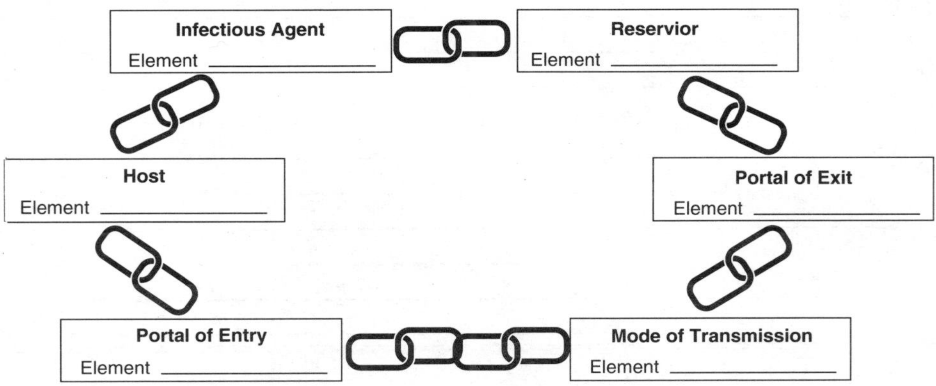

SKIN INTEGRITY

List the **factors** that increase the **risk** of a patient developing a pressure ulcer:

1.____________________
2.____________________
3.____________________
4.____________________
5.____________________
6.____________________
7.____________________
8.____________________
9.____________________
10.____________________
11.____________________

Use the diagram to **circle** the areas of the body where **pressure ulcers** are likely to develop on a bedridden patient:

Case Study: Mrs. Tessie, 88 yrs. old, has been admitted to the hospital for a fractured left elbow. She is malnourished and weighs only 90 lbs. She is currently confused and the physician has ordered a vest posey restraint to prevent her from falling out of bed. Mrs. Tessie has anorexia, her skin is soft and thin. She is incontinent of urine.

Pertinent Terminology	Definition
Pressure ulcer	
Necrosis	
Ischemia	
Reactive hyperemia	
Blanching	
Slough	
Eschar	
Tunneling	
Debridement	
Excoriation	

Use the case study to **circle the number** that best applies to the Mrs. Tessie (the **lower the number**, the greater Mrs. Tessie is at risk for the development of pressure ulcers).

Norton's Pressure Area Risk Assessment Form (Scoring System)

General Physical Condition		Mental State		Activity		Mobility		Incontinence		Total Score
Good	4	Alert	4	Ambulatory	4	Full	4	Absent	4	
Fair	3	Apathetic	3	Walks with help	3	Slightly limited	3	Occasional	3	
Poor	2	Confused	2	Chairbound	2	Very limited	2	Usually urinary	2	
Very bad	1	Stuporous	1	Bedbound	1	Immobile	1	Double	1	______

From Norton, D., McLaren, R., Exton-Smith, AN. *An Investigation of Geriatric Nursing Problems in Hospital.* National Corporation for the Care of Old People (now the Centre for Policy on Ageing), London, 1962. Edinburgh: Churchhill-Livingstone.

» After two days of taking care of Mrs. Tessie, the nurse made the following documentation on the patient's chart: "Reddened, excoriated circular area on sacrum, approximately 2.5 cm by 2.5 cm. Dr. Stanley notified."

» Use the documentation to **check off (✔) the "Stage"** of Mrs. Tessie's pressure ulcer from the **Pressure Ulcer Stages** below:

Stage 1
☐ Nonblanchable erythema of intact skin.

Stage 2
☐ Partial-thickness skin loss involving the epidermis or dermis.

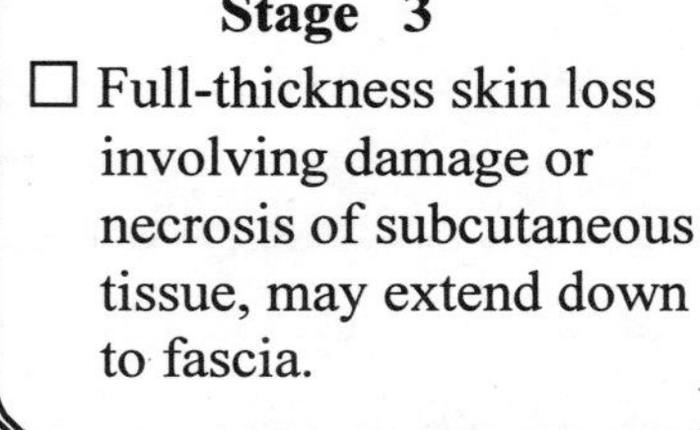

Stage 3
☐ Full-thickness skin loss involving damage or necrosis of subcutaneous tissue, may extend down to fascia.

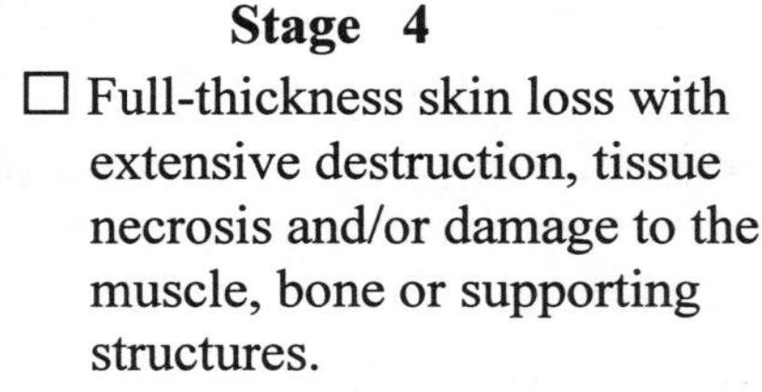

Stage 4
☐ Full-thickness skin loss with extensive destruction, tissue necrosis and/or damage to the muscle, bone or supporting structures.

Interactive Activity: With a partner, **write in** the **"Stage"** of the Pressure Ulcer for each of the following case studies using the **Pressure Ulcer Stages**:

Case Study	Pressure Ulcer Stage
Mr. Hans was found at home unconscious. He has an open wound on his left heel that is 2″ wide and ½″ deep. It has a foul odor and the heel bone is exposed.	______________
The nurse measures an irregular open wound on the right hip. The subcutaneous tissue is visible, but no drainage.	______________

COMMUNICATION

List essential **therapeutic communication techniques** used in a helping relationship:

❖________________ ❖______________

❖________________ ❖______________

❖________________ ❖______________

❖________________ ❖______________

❖________________ ❖______________

Use the diagrams to identify the **factors** that influence communication:

Identify **nontherapeutic responses** that block the development of therapeutic communication:

✷________________________________

✷________________________________

✷________________________________

✷________________________________

✷________________________________

✷________________________________

Case Study: Casey, a student nurse, is in the clinical facility for the first time. She is assigned to Mrs. Reynolds, a 70-yr.-old client, admitted with a fracture of the right hip. Mrs. Reynolds had her own business for 30 years, but is now retired. She remains active in her community. The staff tells Casey that Mrs. Reynolds is a very cranky woman. As soon as Casey walks into the room she hears: "Well, it is about time! If I have to wait any longer I probably would starve to death." Casey responds softly: "I just came on duty."

Pertinent Terminology	Definition
Therapeutic relationship	
Orientation phase	
Testing	
Working phase	
Termination phase	
Paraphrasing	
Open-ended question	

Use the case study to identify **3 factors** that would initially affect the development of a therapeutic relationship with Mrs. Reynolds:

____________________ ____________________ ____________________

Casey's response to Mrs. Reynolds is an example of ✷____________________________

❖ Casey may have addressed Mrs. Reynolds statements by saying:

____

____

Identify the **therapeutic communication technique** used by Casey in the statement and provide a **rationale** as to why this statement is more appropriate:

Therapeutic Technique	Rationale
❖____________________	____________________________
	____________________________

Interactive Activity: With a partner, use the following scenarios to select the appropriate **communication technique** or **response** being utilized:

Paraphrasing   False reassurance   Summarizing

Open-ended question   Clarification   Opinion

1. **Nurse**: "Good morning Mr. Smyth, I heard you had a lot of pain last night. Could you describe the type of pain you had?"______________________________

2. **Family Member**: "The doctor just told me that my husband suffered a severe heart attack!"

   Nurse: "I'm sorry, but don't worry, I'm sure everything will be fine."

   ____

3. **Client**: "I'm just so sick all the time. I just can't do anything by myself anymore. I feel so helpless!"

   Nurse: "It is hard for you to be so dependent and not feel like you are in control. You sound pretty tired of it all."______________________________

4. **Client**: "Nurse, I need to know what pill you gave me this morning."

   Nurse: "Mr. George, I gave you several pills this morning, which one would you like to know more about?" ______________________________

REPORTING PATIENT STATUS

List the most common methods nurse's use to **report patient status** during the shift and from shift to shift:

1.________________________________
2.________________________________
3.________________________________
4.________________________________

Place an "X" in the box(s) that best describes the information that should be included in a **change of shift report**. The change of shift report should:

- ☐ Provide basic information such as room number, date of admission & medical diagnosis
- ☐ Provide specific information regarding the patient needs
- ☐ Provide information on significant changes in the patient's condition
- ☐ Provide information on follow-up patient care.
- ☐ Provide information on patients transferred or discharged from the unit

Case Study: 0700 (morning audiotaped report on the following two patients)
"Mr. Juarez, 76 yrs. old, is in room 461. He was admitted last night with sepsis. He has an IV of D5W infusing at 75 cc/hr. He is NPO. His output for the shift is 150 cc total. The 0600 temperature is 100.6 and his blood pressure is 146/94.

Mr. Henry in room 462 has been here for three days with pneumonia. His temperature at 0600 was 102.4 and I gave him 2 Tylenol tablets. He has an IV infusing at 100 cc/hr and there are 300 cc left. He has a productive cough and is bringing up thick whitish phelgm. I sent the sputum specimen to the laboratory. He has taken in only 50 cc of oral fluid and his output was 275 cc for the shift."

Pertinent Terminology	Definition
Nursing Rand/Kardex	________________________________
	________________________________
Worksheet	________________________________
	________________________________
Reporting	________________________________
	________________________________

Use the **case study** to fill in the worksheet with the pertinent information obtained in the morning report on the two patients:

Worksheet

Pt. Name:____________ Age:____________ VS____________ Amb. ______ Bedrest____ Bath (self)____ (Bed)____	Rm: _____ I = _____ O= _____ Diet:_____	Dx:________ Admit date:_____ IV:________ ________ ________	Follow-up Notes: ________ ________ ________ ________
Pt. Name:____________ Age:____________ VS____________ Amb. ______ Bedrest____ Bath (self)____ (Bed)____	Rm: _____ I = _____ O= _____ Diet:_____	Dx:________ Admit date:_____ IV:________ ________ ________	Follow-up Notes: ________ ________ ________ ________

Additional information to **complete the worksheet is found** in the ____________________.

Interactive Activity: With a partner, answer the questions regarding (1) the **change of shift report** for the following case study and (2) **fill in the worksheet** and discuss the **Follow-up Notes**:

1500 (**change of shift** audiotaped report)
"Mr. Warren Taylor, 92 yrs. old, in room 357 was admitted yesterday with anemia. His hemoglobin (Hgb) this morning is 7.2 mg/dL and his hematocrit (Hct) is 26%. He is hard of hearing and weighs 117 lbs. His Foley drained only 100 cc all shift. He has an IV of Normal Saline infusing at 75 cc/hr. He will receive two units of blood this evening. The lab will call when the blood is ready. The family and the patient will make a decision soon regarding his code status. He is very weak and needs a lot of assistance."

☞**Identify the basic information** given in the report: ____________________________

____

☞**Identify the significant information** given in the report: ________________________

____

Worksheet

Pt. Name:____________ **Age:**____________ **VS:**____________ **Amb.** ______ **Bedrest**____ **Bath (self)**____ **(Bed)**____	**Rm:** _____ **I =** _____ **O=** _____ **Diet:**_____	**Dx:**________ **Admit date:**_____ **IV:**________ ________ ________	**Follow-up Notes:** ________ ________ ________ ________ ________

INTRODUCTION TO THE ASSESSMENT PROCESS

List the **methods** available to the nurse for the **collection of patient data**:

1.______________________________
2.______________________________
3.______________________________
4.______________________________

List the **parts of the Patient's Chart** that assist the nurse in the **collection of patient data**:

1.______________________________
2.______________________________
3.______________________________
4.______________________________
5.______________________________
6.______________________________

Draw a line to connect all the **Objective Data**.

Subjective Data

"I have a headache"

Gold colored Chain

States Nauseated

Resp. 22 Regular

WBC 5,000 mm today

Objective Data

Case Study: Mrs. Clark has been admitted to the hospital for the birth of her baby. Her husband is by her side. You observe that she is very pleasant but cries out with each contraction. She tells you "I feel a lot of pressure in my back." Her chart indicates that she is 26 yrs. old and that she has a 6-yr.-old son.

Pertinent Terminology	Definition
Assessment	
Subjective data	
Objective data	
Clustering data	
Validation of data	
Primary source	
Secondary source	

Use the case study to identify the following information:

Source
(Primary/Secondary)

✎ List the **objective data**:

✎ List the **subjective data**:

Interactive Activity: With a partner, **use the box to identify the subjective and objective data** from the case studies:

§ Mrs. Toby has been admitted with depression. She answers questions, softly,with a "yes" or "no" response. She wants her door closed and her room dark. She refuses visitors and only eats 10% of her meals. You noticed that she cries regularly and sleeps a lot. She bites her nails frequently.

Objective data
Subjective data

§ Mr. Peale had surgery one day ago. He tells you that he has been very independent all his life and hates being sick. He has refused his pain medication all morning. You notice that he refuses to get out of bed, he moans quietly every now and then, he is sweaty and his hands are clenched tightly. His surgical dressing is clean and he says everything is fine when you ask him a question.

Objective data
Subjective data

§ Mr. Keil informs the nursing assistant that he is nauseated. He has refused his lunch. You go in to check him and you notice 100 cc of clear yellow emesis. He tells you that he vomited. His wife is at his bedside.

Objective data
Subjective data

BASIC PHYSICAL ASSESSMENT

List the **four methods of examination** used in the performance of a physical assessment:

1.____________________________

2.____________________________

3.____________________________

4.____________________________

Write-in the most appropriate **method of examination(s)** for each of the following:

- ♦ Oral mucous membranes ____________________________
- ♦ Peripheral pulses ____________________________
- ♦ Arterial blood pressure ____________________________
- ♦ Lung sounds ____________________________
- ♦ Lower extremity edema ____________________________
- ♦ Apical pulse ____________________________
- ♦ Distended abdomen ____________________________

Case Study: Carrie is a nursing student who is assigned to Ms. Waldron. Ms. Waldron, 18 yrs. old, came in to the ER complaining of right lower abdominal pains. She had an appendectomy 2 days ago and will be going home this afternoon. Carrie performs a **body systems assessment** and documents the following notes:
Neuro: Alert and oriented x3. **Cardiovascular (CV)**: Radial pulse regular and bounding. **Skin**: warm and dry, pallor present, turgor elastic. **Respirations (Resp.)**: Regular, clear. **Gastrointestinal (GI)**: Bowel sounds present in all four quadrants. RLQ abdominal dressing clean, complains of tenderness c̄ palpation. **Genitourinary (GU)**: States voiding without difficulty. **Musculoskeletal (MS)**: Ambulates with a steady gait. **Psychosocial**: Cheerful.

Pertinent Terminology	Definition
Inspection	
Palpation	
Percussion	
Chief Complaint (CC)	
Review of Systems	

Use the documentation notes from the case study to **identify the method of examination** used by Carrie in performing the body systems assessment:

Documentation	Method(s) of Examination
♦ **Neuro**: Alert and oriented **x3**	______________
♦ **CV**: Radial pulse regular and bounding	______________
♦ **Skin**: Warm and dry, pallor present, turgor elastic	______________ ______________
♦ **Resp**.: Regular, clear	______________
♦ **GI**: Bowel sounds present in all four quadrants. RLQ abdominal dressing clean complains of tenderness c̄ palpation	______________
♦ **GU**: States voiding without difficulty	______________
♦ **MS**: Ambulates with a steady gait	______________
♦ **Psychosocial**: Cheerful	______________

Interactive Activity: With a partner, use the following documentation notes to **(1) identify** the **body system** being assessed and **(2) the method of examination** used:

Documentation Notes	♦ Body System/Method(s) of Examination
States it is 1945, does not know where he is at. Knows first name. Hand grips unequal right < left.	♦ ______________ ______________
Voided 50 cc of amber fluid. Abdomen distended.	♦ ______________ ______________
Warm, moist. Pallor with erythema on sacral area. Edema 1+ on bilateral lower extemeties.	♦ ______________ ______________
Absent bowel sounds in lower and upper right quadrants, hyperactive on upper and lower left quadrant. Having small amounts of liquid dark brown stools.	♦ ______________ ______________
Wheezes audible on inspiration, coughing, expectorating thick yellowish phelgm.	♦ ______________ ______________
Apical pulse 116, rapid, irregular. Radial pulse 98, rapid, thready, irregular	♦ ______________ ______________
Passive ROM to right hand. Unable to extend and flex fingers.	♦ ______________ ______________
Left facial drooping. Left arm and leg flaccid.	♦ ______________ ______________

SELF-CONCEPT

List the **four components** of **self-concept**:

1.________________________

2.________________________

3.________________________

4.________________________

For each of the **self-concept** components **identify 2 stressors** that affect and contribute to altering the component of:

- **Identity**
  ____
  ____
- **Body image**
  ____
  ____
- **Self-esteem**
  ____
  ____
- **Role performance**
  ____
  ____

Case Study: Mrs. Mathews was diagnosed with breast cancer 2 weeks ago and had a left mastectomy. She is 32 yrs. old, married with a 5 yr. old daughter. She is very anxious after the surgery and wonders how her husband will react to her. She tells the nurse: "I am so young to have this done." She begins to cry and says that she loves being a mom, but doesn't think she can have another child because she would not be able to nurse and care for the baby as she would like to. She is scheduled to begin chemotherapy treatments in 1 week.

Pertinent Terminology	Definition
Self-concept	
Identity	
Body image	
Self-esteem	
Role performance	

Reread the case study and cluster the **objective data** and **subjective data** that relate to the **self-concept** component that is marked with an “**X**”:

- ☐ Identity
- ☒ **Body image**
- ☐ Self-esteem
- ☐ Role performance

➔ **Objective data:**

➔ **Subjective data:**

- ☐ Identity
- ☐ Body image
- ☐ Self-esteem
- ☒ **Role performance**

➔ **Objective data:**

➔ **Subjective data:**

Interactive Activity: With a partner, use the following case study to cluster the objective data and the subjective data related to the **self-concept** component that is marked with an “**X**”:

CASE STUDY

Mr. Jenkins suffered a heart attack 2 months ago and has lost his job. When he comes to the clinic, his facial expression is tense and he speaks in a hostile voice. During the last visit, he stated: “I can’t just sit here, I am the breadwinner of my family.” “I’m useless since I had the heart attack!”

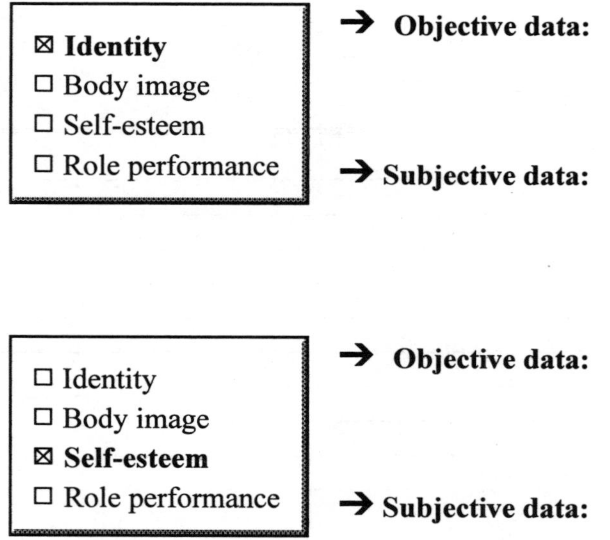

CULTURAL ASPECTS OF NURSING

List the **six cultural phenomena** that influence nursing care:

1.______________________________
2.______________________________
3.______________________________
4.______________________________
5.______________________________
6.______________________________

List **2 examples** for each of the following:

❄ **Communication**
1.______________________
2.______________________

❄ **Social organizations**
1.______________________
2.______________________

❄ **Environmental control**
1.______________________
2.______________________

❄ **Biological variations**
1.______________________
2.______________________

Case Study: Wendy RN, the home health nurse, visits Mrs. Fuentes, a 62-yr.-old Hispanic woman who has had diabetes mellitus for twenty years and currently has a sore on her left foot. Mrs. Fuentes has missed two of her doctor's appointments and has been soaking her foot in warm salt water every night. Mrs. Fuentes speaks English but does not like to bother anyone. She enjoys cooking and eating Mexican food. During the home visit, Wendy noticed several religious artifacts and many pictures of her children and grandchildren.

Pertinent Terminology	Definition
Culture	
Culture shock	
Cultural sensitivity	
Ethnicity	
Acculturation	
Ethnocentrism	
Transcultural nursing	

Use the case study to **identify** the **cultural data** that relates to the **culture phenomena** listed below:

Culture phenomena	Cultural data
❊ Communication	________________
❊ Space	________________
❊ Time	________________
❊ Social organization	________________
❊ Environmental control	________________
❊ Biological variations	________________

Interactive Activity: With a partner, use the following case studies to (1) **underline** the pertinent **cultural data** and (2) **identify** the **possible implications** for health care delivery:

Case Study	Health Care Delivery Implication(s)
Mrs. Paredes, a Filipino woman, is a very quiet patient. She rarely complains and nurses comment on how she doesn't maintain eye contact when the nurse is talking.	________________
Mrs. Lee, a patient of Chinese ancestry, is 80 yrs. old and requires constant care. She lives with one of her daughters and the family members take turns caring for her at night.	________________
Mrs. Wright has had a miscarriage. She hemorrhaged and her blood count is very low. The physician has recommended a blood transfusion, but Mrs. Wright refuses because of her religious beliefs.	________________
Mrs. James is an African-American woman, a widow, who comes to the outpatient clinic for blood pressure checks. She tells the nurse that her youngest daughter is about to be married. She is concerned because her other daughter has sickle cell anemia.	________________
Mr. Clarke had major surgery yesterday. He does not want to get out of bed and has refused all his pain medication. The nurse knows that he is in pain, but wants to respect his wishes.	________________

INTRODUCTION TO FORMULATING A NURSING DIAGNOSIS

List the **5 steps of the Nursing Process**:

1.______________________________
2.______________________________
3.______________________________
4.______________________________
5.______________________________

The **NANDA Nursing Diagnoses** are classified and formulated to address the patient's health problems which can be:

1.______________________________
2.______________________________
3.______________________________
4.______________________________

Circle the **words** that may be used to give specific meaning to the Nursing Diagnosis statement:

Related to
Increased
Well
Altered
High Risk
Acute
Impaired
Sign/symptom
Due to
Possible

Case Study: Judy, the Home Health nurse makes the following observations and documents the following after visiting Mr. Toby: Mr. Toby lives alone, his only son lives 60 miles away, visits monthly and calls weekly. Mr. Toby stays indoors all day. His vision is poor and he is not able to drive.

Pertinent Terminology	Definition
NANDA	
Nursing Process	
Assessment	
Nursing Diagnosis	
Defining Characteristics	
Planning	
Implementation	
Evaluation	
Etiology	

From the case study, **check off (✓) the Nursing Diagnosis** most appropriate for Mr. Toby (✳ Use a Nursing Diagnosis book to validate your selection):

Nursing Diagnoses:

_____ Ineffective coping
_____ Risk for loneliness
_____ Social isolation

List the **defining characteristics** for the **nursing diagnosis** you selected:

✳_______________ ✳_______________ ✳_______________

✳_______________ ✳_______________

☞ **Further documentation** by the home health nurse states: Mr. Toby has lost 10 lbs. since the last visit—two weeks ago. He now is malnourished. Mr. Toby is on a limited income. He needs the services of a nutritionist and a community service that delivers meals to homebound individuals.

From the **further documentation** data, **check off (✓) the Nursing Diagnosis** most appropriate for Mr. Toby:

Nursing Diagnoses:

_____ Social isolation
_____ Knowledge deficit
_____ Altered nutrition: less than body requirements

List the **current pertinent defining characteristics** for the nursing diagnosis you selected:

✳_______________ ✳_______________ ✳_______________

Interactive Activity: With a partner, review the following case studies and **identify** the **defining characteristics** that relate to the **Nursing Diagnosis** written next to each situation:

Case Study	✳ Defining Characteristics
Mrs. Shaw has a Stage II pressure ulcer on her right heel. She has been on bedrest and her right leg is elevated.	Impaired skin integrity: actual ✳_______________
Mr. Clarke has oral lesions in his mouth caused by a treatment of chemotherapy. He complains of pain and his mouth is red.	Altered oral mucous membranes ✳_______________
Mrs. Morning-Star is scheduled for surgery in the morning. She says that she is very scared because her grandmother died having surgery.	Fear ✳_______________

FORMULATING A NURSING DIAGNOSIS

List the components of the:

Two-part Nursing Diagnosis statement:

1.________________________________

2.________________________________

Three-part Nursing Diagnosis statement:

1.________________________________

2.________________________________

3.________________________________

Place an "X" in the box that identifies the common **errors** made in the development of the Nursing Diagnosis statement:

- ☐ Using the NANDA diagnostic categories to identify the nursing diagnosis
- ☐ Using the medical diagnosis in the formulation of the nursing diagnosis
- ☐ Clustering the subjective/objective data
- ☐ Using signs and symptoms to write the nursing diagnosis statement
- ☐ Making legally inadvisable statements
- ☐ Misinterpreting the meaning of the subjective and objective data
- ☐ Being very specific in defining the etiology
- ☐ Using qualifying words in the diagnostic statement

Case Study: Ms. Telly is to be scheduled for elective surgery. In preparation for the surgery, the office nurse takes Ms. Telly's health history. The nurse documents that Ms. Telly has recently been diagnosed with Diabetes Mellitus and was prescribed an antidiabetic pill to take every morning. Ms. Telly tells the nurse that she stopped the "pill" one week ago because she was feeling better.

Pertinent Terminology	Definition
Nursing diagnosis	
Defining characteristics	
Risk factors	
Etiology	
Data cluster	

Use the case study to **identify** the **cultural data** that relates to the **culture phenomena** listed below:

Culture phenomena	Cultural data
✻ Communication	____________
✻ Space	____________
✻ Time	____________
✻ Social organization	____________
✻ Environmental control	____________
✻ Biological variations	____________

Interactive Activity: With a partner, use the following case studies to (1) **underline** the pertinent **cultural data** and (2) **identify** the **possible implications** for health care delivery:

Case Study	Health Care Delivery Implication(s)
Mrs. Paredes, a Filipino woman, is a very quiet patient. She rarely complains and nurses comment on how she doesn't maintain eye contact when the nurse is talking.	____________
Mrs. Lee, a patient of Chinese ancestry, is 80 yrs. old and requires constant care. She lives with one of her daughters and the family members take turns caring for her at night.	____________
Mrs. Wright has had a miscarriage. She hemorrhaged and her blood count is very low. The physician has recommended a blood transfusion, but Mrs. Wright refuses because of her religious beliefs.	____________
Mrs. James is an African-American woman, a widow, who comes to the outpatient clinic for blood pressure checks. She tells the nurse that her youngest daughter is about to be married. She is concerned because her other daughter has sickle cell anemia.	____________
Mr. Clarke had major surgery yesterday. He does not want to get out of bed and has refused all his pain medication. The nurse knows that he is in pain, but wants to respect his wishes.	____________

ASSESSMENT OF THE ELDERLY PATIENT

List the **interventions** that would assist in communicating with an elderly patient who is experiencing hearing loss related to the aging process:

1.______________________________

2.______________________________

3.______________________________

4.______________________________

5.______________________________

List the **interventions** that would assist in an elderly patient who is experiencing vision problems related to the aging process:

1.______________________________

2.______________________________

3.______________________________

4.______________________________

5.______________________________

Mark an **"X"** in the appropriate column that identifies the effects of aging on the following:

	Decreased	**Increased**
Sensory perception	☐	☐
Visual acuity	☐	☐
Gag reflex	☐	☐
Skin tissue elasticity	☐	☐
Body temperature	☐	☐
Cardiac output	☐	☐
RBC production	☐	☐
Plasma viscosity	☐	☐
Lung capacity	☐	☐
Residual urine	☐	☐

Case Study: The following information was been given to a group of students regarding the assessment of a elderly patient: Responds slowly, but appropriately to all questions, skin warm, dry, thin, and flaky. Skin turgor >3 secs. Capillary refill >3 secs. Respirations short and shallow, lung sounds with bilateral crackles. 50% intake, states food is very bland. BM this morning moderate amount formed hard stool. Bilateral lower extremities with 1+ pitting edema. Toenails yellowish, thick. Vital signs T. 99, P. 84, R. 16, BP 160/80.

Pertinent Terminology	Definition
Arcus senilis	
Edema	
Pitting edema	
Kyphosis	
Presbycusis	
Turgor	

Use the information from the case study below to mark an "**X**" on the data that is representative of the normal effects of the aging process:

_____Responds slowly, but appropriately to all questions

_____Skin warm, dry, thin, and flaky

_____Skin turgor >3 secs. Capillary refill >3 secs

_____Respirations short and shallow, lung sounds with bilateral crackles

_____50% intake, states food is very bland

_____BM this morning formed hard stool

_____Bilateral lower extremities with 1+ pitting edema.

_____Toenails yellowish, thick

_____Vital signs T. 99, P. 84, R. 16, BP 160/80

Interactive Activity: With a partner, use the information provided to **(1) underline** the assessment data that represents the **effects of the normal aging process** and **(2) select** the NANDA Nursing Diagnosis most appropriate for the situation:

ASSESSMENT DATA	NURSING DIAGNOSIS
Wife in to see patient, states that husband is confused this morning, does not know that he is in the hospital. Further patient assessment, PERRLA, whitish ring noted around the margins of the iris, uses glasses. Mouth dry, wears upper dentures.	☐ Altered thought processes ☐ Altered mucous membrane ☐ Acute confusion ☐ Impaired memory
Skin pale, translucent. Lower extremities thin, pedal pulses weak, palpable. States has loss of a small amount of urine when coughs. Shortness of breath, R 28, mouth breathing. Abdomen round, soft, nontender. Temp. 96.8.	☐ Functional incontinence ☐ Hypothermia ☐ Altered peripheral tissue perfusion ☐ Ineffective breathing pattern
Transfers independently out of bed, complained of dizziness when coming to a standing position, gait slow. Anterior-posterior diameter of chest increased. Soft diet, intake 70%	☐ Impaired physical mobility ☐ Risk for injury ☐ Altered health maintenance ☐ Altered nutrition, less than body requirements

CARING FOR THE SURGICAL PATIENT

List the **two major** types of anesthesia:

1.____________________________

2.____________________________

List the **types of regional anesthesia**:

1.____________________________

2.____________________________

3.____________________________

4.____________________________

5.____________________________

Identify into which of the perioperative phases **(preoperative, intraoperative, postoperative)** the following interventions would be started:

	Pre	**Intra**	**Post**
Use of incentive inspirometer	☐	☐	☐
Coughing and deep breathing	☐	☐	☐
Splinting of surgical site	☐	☐	☐
Prepping surgical site	☐	☐	☐
Changing the surgical dressing	☐	☐	☐
Leg exercises	☐	☐	☐
Pain management	☐	☐	☐
Discharge instructions	☐	☐	☐

Case Study: Mrs. Hale is admitted for a total abdominal hysterectomy (TAH) this morning. She is 52 yrs. old and is obese. Her past medical history indicates that she stopped smoking 5 years ago. Both parents are deceased. Mother died at the age of 88 and father died from a heart attack at the age of 62. Mrs. Hale's vital signs are: T. 97.8 - P. 76 - R. 18 BP 164/92. The following laboratory studies were done: CBC, PT, serum electrolytes of Na^+, K^+, serum FBS, BUN and creatinine, UA. Chest x-ray report and ECG are in the chart.

Pertinent Terminology	**Definition**
General anesthesia	
Regional anesthesia	
Thrombophlebitis	
Atelectasis	
Paralytic ileus	
PCA	
Pneumatic compression device	

From the case study, **list** the factors that increase Mrs. Hale's risk of postop complications:

* ______________________ * ______________________

* ______________________ * ______________________

Interactive Activity: With a partner, use the follow-up case study to **(1) identify** which medical order the nurse would do **first** and **(2) list the priority nursing interventions** the nurse would **independently perform** and provide a **rationale** for each intervention:

Follow-up case study: Mrs. Hale returns from the Post Anesthesia Room (PAR), sleepy but easily arousable. The physician writes the following postop orders:

NPO - May have sips of water in the AM
IV - 5% Dextrose/0.9 % Normal Saline infuse at 100 cc/hr
Ambulate this evening
VS q30 min for first hour, then q1h x2 hrs, then q4 hrs
Incentive spirometer q1h while awake
PCA - Morphine sulfate set at 1 mg/6min (not to exceed 30 mg/4 hrs)
Antiembolic stocking and pneumatic compression device to legs continuously
Indwelling urinary catheter to gravity—remove in AM

First Medical Orders to Implement	Rationale

Priority Independent Nursing Interventions	Rationale

WOUND ASSESSMENT

List the **types of wounds**:

1.______________________________

2.______________________________

List the **types of wound drainage** systems:

1.______________________________

2.______________________________

3.______________________________

Match the **wound classifications and wound drainage terminology** with the appropriate description or characteristics:

1. Laceration	___ Thin, clear watery secretion
2. Contusion	___ Containing pus
3. Penetrating	___ Open cut made with a knife/scalpel
4. Abrasion	___ Containing RBCs
5. Incision	___ Irregular wound tear; jagged edges
6. Serosanguinous	___ Entering into the tissues/body cavity
7. Serous	___ Closed wound; with pain, swelling, & discoloration
8. Sanguinous	___ Red, watery secretion
9. Purulent	___ A scraping away of the skin surface

Case Study: Mr. Jenkins, 26 yrs. old, received a stab wound to his abdomen and was taken to the Emergency Room. He underwent emergency surgery. He has an IV, nasogastric tube to continuous low wall suction and one Jackson-Pratt on the RUQ and another on the LLQ of the abdomen. He has a closed abdominal wound and the dressing is clean and dry as he is taken to the surgical unit at 0800.

Pertinent Terminology	**Definition**
Primary intention	
Tertiary intention	
Secondary intention	
Granulation tissue	
Inflammatory phase	
Maturation phase	
Proliferation phase	
Dehiscence	
Evisceration	

Use the case study to **check off (✓)** all the factors that apply to Mr. Jenkins:

☐ High risk for infection	☐ Postoperative pain should initially increase
☐ Healing by secondary intention	☐ J-P drainage should progressively decrease
☐ J-P will aid in the healing process	☐ Slight redness around incision first day

✘ Three hours after arriving on the surgical unit, the nurse took the vital signs and noted that Mr. Jenkin's surgical dressing has two abd pads and is currently saturated with sanguinous drainage. The nurse lightly palpated the abdomen.

Abdominal Surgical Dressing

Implement the appropriate nursing interventions on the adbominal surgical dressing:

✘ **Select** the nurse's documentation that demonstrates the appropriate assessment:

____ Abdominal dressing c̄ large amount of red drainage, abdomen tender. T 100.4

____ Abdominal dressing covered c̄ pink reddish drainage, abdomen tender, no bowel sounds. P. 88 BP 136/86.

____ Abdominal dressing saturated c̄ red drainage, abdomen tender, reinforced. P. 88 BP 136/86.

Interactive Activity: With a partner, use the **statements** below to **(1) check off (✓)** whether the statement is correct or incorrect and **(2)** provide a rationale for your selection.

Statements	Correct/Incorrect	Rationale
1. Wound drainage devices need to be emptied once a shift	☐ Correct ☐ Incorrect	
2. Wound drainage devices need to be compressed to function	☐ Correct ☐ Incorrect	
3. Assessment of the wound should be done once a day	☐ Correct ☐ Incorrect	
4. Wound description does not need to include wound measurement	☐ Correct ☐ Incorrect	
5. Wound evisceration requires the application of sterile dry gauze	☐ Correct ☐ Incorrect	

THE PATIENT WITH FLUID & ELECTROLYTE IMBALANCE

List the **adult normal values** for the following electrolytes:

1. Sodium (Na^+) = ____________
2. Potassium (K^+) = ____________
3. Chloride (Cl^-) = ____________
4. Calcium (Ca^{2+}) = ____________
5. Phosphate (PO_4^-) = ____________
6. Magnesium (Mg^{2+}) = ____________

Write in the appropriate medical terminology for the serum laboratory values below:

Mg^{2+} 3.5 mg/dl = ____________

K^+ 2.5 mEq/L = ____________

Cl^- 90 mEq/L = ____________

Na^+ 132 mEq/L = ____________

Ca^{2+} 8.5 mg/dl = ____________

PO_4^- 5.1 mg/dl = ____________

Case Study: Mr. Howard, 36 yrs. old, was admitted with gastroenteritis. He has been vomiting and having severe diarrhea for two days. He is very weak. The current lab results are: Na^+ 128 mEq/L, K^+ 2.8 mEq/L, Cl^- 90 mEq/L. The physician orders IV of 0.9% NS at 100 cc/hr, NPO and I & O.

Pertinent Terminology	Definition
Sodium (Na^+)	
Potassium (K^+)	
Chloride (Cl^-)	
Calcium (Ca^{2+})	
Phosphate (PO_4^-)	
Magnesium (Mg^{2+})	
Third space syndrome	
Edema	
Pitting edema	

From the case study, identify the abnormal laboratory results. List the **major clinical signs or symptoms** that you would assess with each abnormal value:

* ______________ = ______________________________________
____
____

* ______________ = ______________________________________
____
____

* ______________ = ______________________________________
____
____

☞ **Follow-up case study:** Mr. Howard's vomiting and diarrhea has begun to subside in the evening and the M.D. has ordered a clear liquid diet. Mr. Howard's **24 hour Intake and Output** for the day is charted below:

24 Hour Intake/Output Record

Intake	Output
IV = 2400 Oral = 120	Emesis = 950 Diarrhea = 900 Urine = 750
2520 cc	2600 cc

☞ Based on the case study and Intake and Output Record **select** the most appropriate **NANDA Nursing Diagnoses** for Mr. Howard:

____ Fluid volume excess
____ Diarrhea
____ Altered nutrition: Less than body requirements
____ Fluid volume deficit
____ Impaired skin integrity
____ Risk for injury

Interactive Activity: With a partner, read the case study below and write a **rationale** for each of the nursing interventions listed:

Case Study	Nursing Interventions	Rationale
Sallie May was admitted with heart failure. The nursing diagnosis of "Fluid volume excess r/t noncompliance to dietary Na^+ restriction" is listed in her NCP. Digoxin 0.25 mg qd po, furosemide 40 mg qd po, and K-Dur 10 mEq po tid are her medications.	▸ Weigh daily ▸ Monitor I & O ▸ Take apical pulse ▸ Assess skin ▸ Assess lungs ▸ ✓Neck veins	

ELIMINATION - URINARY

List the **factors** that affect bladder elimination:

1.________________________________
2.________________________________
3.________________________________
4.________________________________
5.________________________________
6.________________________________
7.________________________________
8.________________________________
9.________________________________

Use the diagrams to **select** the appropriate size of the indwelling catheter for the female and male patient. **Draw a line** on the catheter at the anticipated length of insertion.

Female

14 fr

18 fr

Male

20 fr

16 fr

Case Study: Mrs. Sunn, 42 yrs. old, had abdominal surgery two days ago. She has an IV infusing into her left forearm, an indwelling urinary catheter (Foley) and she has a temperature of 100.4°F this evening. The physician orders the indwelling catheter to be removed in the AM.

Pertinent Terminology	Definition
UA	
Nocturia	
Hematuria	
Dysuria	
Oliguria	
Anuria	
Urinary incontinence	
Residual urine	
Midstream UA	
Void	
Indwelling catheter	
Condom catheter	

Using the information in the case study, the nurse gathers more information and documents on Mrs. Sunn's chart. **Select the statement** below which describes a thorough observation of the urinary system:

1. Indwelling catheter patent to gravity. Taking fluids liberally.
2. Indwelling catheter to gravity, draining cloudy pale yellow urine.
3. Indwelling catheter patent to gravity, output 75 cc.
4. Indwelling catheter patent, draining freely. Abdomen without distention.

✓ The next morning, the nurse prepares to remove the indwelling catheter. Identify the equipment the nurse needs to gather to properly remove the catheter.

____

✓✓ The indwelling catheter is removed at 0800. The nurse knows that Mrs. Sunn should void within __________ hours after the removal of the catheter.

Interactive Activity: With a partner, **select the NANDA Nursing Diagnosis** that is most appropriate to the case studies below that describe the complications Mrs. Sunn experienced after the removal of the indwelling catheter.

NANDA Nursing Diagnosis:
(1) Stress incontinence
(2) Urinary retention
(3) Altered urinary elimination
(4) Risk for infection

Case Study	Nursing Diagnosis
Mrs. Sunn is unable to void 8 hours after the removal of the indwelling catheter. She is experiencing abdominal discomfort, a sensation of fullness and frequent dribbling.	____________
Mrs. Sunn is catheterized for residual urine and 700 cc of urine are drained from the bladder. An indwelling catheter is left in place.	____________
The following day the catheter is removed. Mrs. Sunn is able to void without any further problems that day. The next day she complains of dysuria and hematuria when she voids.	____________
Mrs. Sunn is started on an antibiotic. She notices that the dysuria and hematuria are no longer present. However she tells you that she has a history of losing urine when she coughs or sneezes.	____________

ELIMINATION - BOWEL

List the **factors** that affect bowel elimination:

1.____________________
2.____________________
3.____________________
4.____________________
5.____________________
6.____________________
7.____________________

Use the diagram to identify the location and placement of the stethoscope when listening for bowel sounds. Draw a **circle** at each location.

Case Study: The M.D. writes the following on the History and Physical form after examining Mr. Casey Miller, 55 yrs. old: Complains of cramping abdominal pain, borborygmi, 5-6 dark brown semi-liquid BMs/day for several days. Last bowel movement this AM. Indicates no changes in diet intake. Denies melena, constipation, nausea, or vomiting. The M.D. orders an Endoscopy, Barium Enema, and stool sample for occult blood.

Pertinent Terminology	Definition
Bowel sounds	
Flatus	
Constipation	
Diarrhea	
Occult blood	
Melena	
Enema	
Fecal impaction	
Borborygmi	
Endoscopy	
Barium enema	

Using the information identified in the History and Physical, identify the questions that the nurse could ask Mr. Miller in order to **assess** the bowel pattern changes that he is currently experiencing:

1. Complains of cramping abdominal pain, borborygmi.
Question: ____________________

2. 5-6 dark brown semi-liquid BMs/day for several days.
Question: ____________________

3. Indicates no changes in diet intake.
Question: ____________________

4. Denies melena, constipation, nausea, or vomiting.
Question: ____________________

5. Last bowel movement this AM.
Question: ____________________

Write **2** questions that would be useful in further assessing Mr. Casey Miller's bowel function:
1.____________________

2.____________________

Discuss how these questions contribute to the assessment.

Interactive Activity: With a partner, select the **NANDA Nursing Diagnosis** that best applies to each of the case scenarios below:

NANDA Nursing Diagnosis: (1) Perceived Constipation (2) Diarrhea (3) Colonic Constipation (4) Bowel Incontinence

Case Study	Nursing Diagnosis
Mr. Bay takes a mild laxative every night since his retirement one year ago. He believes that his change in activity will cause him bowel problems.	____________
Mrs. Clariz was in a car accident one month ago in which she sustained a neuromuscular back injury. While hospitalized she was having involuntary frequent loose BMs.	____________
The Nursing Diagnosis for Mr. Casey Miller is	____________

GENERAL NUTRITION

List the **four therapeutic diets** commonly encountered in the clinical setting (exclude the special diets):

1.______________________________
2.______________________________
3.______________________________
4.______________________________

List the most common methods of providing enteral nutrition:

1.______________________________
2.______________________________
3.______________________________
4.______________________________

Draw a line to connect the following **foods** with the appropriate **common therapeutic diets** encountered in the clinical setting:

Clear Liquid

Soft

Full Liquid

Ice cream
Carbonated beverages
Broth fat-free
Cooked vegetables
Cream of rice
Puddings
Smooth peanut butter
Clear fruit juices
Bananas
Custard
Sherbert
Eggs

Case Study: Mr. Grier, 68 yrs. old, had a cerebral vascular accident (CVA) two weeks ago. He has right-sided hemiplegia. The nursing care rand indicates that Mr. Grier is on a soft, pureed diet and is on Intake and Output.

Pertinent Terminology	Definition
Regular diet	
Soft diet	
Full liquid	
Clear liquid	
Enteral nutrition	
Gastric lavage	
Gastrostomy tube	
PEG	
Jejunostomy tube	

Use the information from the case study to **mark an "X"** on the most appropriate feeding guidelines for Mr. Grier who has right-sided hemiplegia:

Feeding Guidelines

- ☐ Give water frequently with the food
- ☐ Place in high Fowler's position
- ☐ Check right cheek for "pocketing"
- ☐ Give thickened juices
- ☐ Place in semi-Fowler's position
- ☐ Provide finger foods
- ☐ Allow family to feed Mr. Grier
- ☐ Lie flat after feeding

Interactive Activity: With a partner, use the case studies related to Mr. Grier. For each situation **prioritize the NANDA Nursing Diagnosis**, **#1** = Highest priority, **#2** = Important, and **#3** = Need to monitor.

Case Study	NANDA Nursing Diagnosis
Mr. Grier's intake for last 24 hrs = 1250cc and his output = 725cc. He is fatigued and needs to be reminded to drink and eat. His skin is dry and flaky. Skin turgor-tenting. Oral mucous membranes dry, teeth missing. Urine color is dark yellow.	____ Fluid volume deficit r/t decreased fluid intake secondary to fatigue ____ Risk for altered oral mucous membranes r/t insufficient intake of fluids ____ Risk for impaired skin integrity r/t dry, thin skin secondary to aging
Mr. Grier began to cough forcefully while being fed. The feeding was stopped and the M.D. ordered for him to be NPO. Mr. Grier has lost 3 lbs in one week. He has an IV of D5W infusing at 75 cc/hr. It is difficult to get him out of bed, since he is weak and does not assist in the transfer.	____ Altered nutrition r/t weakness, fatigue, and NPO status ____ Risk for aspiration r/t impaired swallowing ____ Risk for impaired skin integrity r/t prolonged bedrest

GASTROINTESTINAL

List the structures in the gastrointestinal tract involved with the digestion and absorption of food:

1.__________________________

2.__________________________

3.__________________________

4.__________________________

5.__________________________

Use the diagram to **identify the quadrants** (RLQ, RUQ, LLQ, LUQ) and the **anatomical regions of the abdomen** (Right and Left Lumbar, Right and Left Inguinal, Umbilical, Epigastric, Suprapubic, and Right and Left Hypochondriac)

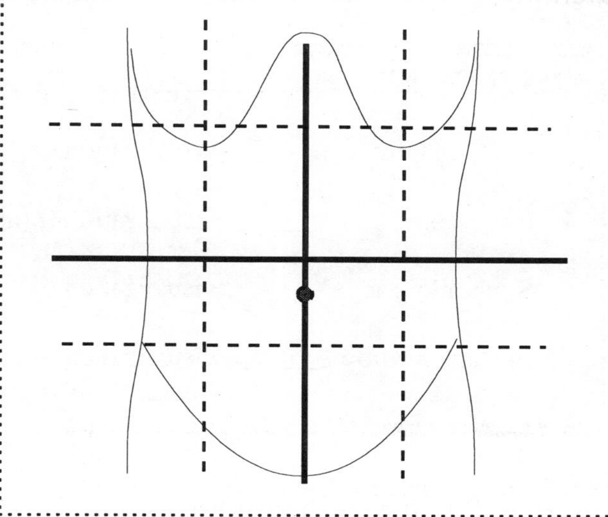

Modified from Black, J.M., Matassarin-Jacobs, E. (1997). *Medical-Surgical Nursing: Clinical Management for Continuity of Care* (5th ed). Philadelphia: W.B. Saunders Co., p. 1708.

Case Study: Mrs. Tripp is a 55-year-old woman who was admitted to the hospital with complaints of diarrhea for the past ten days. She states that she has abdominal cramping and at times passes bloody stools. She is scheduled for a colonoscopy at 10:00 AM today.

Pertinent Terminology	Definition
Duodenum	
Jejunum	
Ileum	
Cecum	
Colon	
Rectum	
Polyp	

Use the case study to **(✓) check off all the nursing interventions and physician's orders** that you would associate with the preparation of Mrs. Tripp for the colonoscopy procedure.

- ☐ NPO for procedure
- ☐ GoLYTELY is given for stool evacuation
- ☐ Monitor for abdominal pain and bleeding postprocedure
- ☐ Consent is necessary
- ☐ May have a clear liquid breakfast
- ☐ Requires general anesthesia

Match the gastrointestinal diagnostic tests with the appropriate definitions:

DIAGNOSTIC TESTS		DEFINITIONS
1. Colonoscopy	_______	visualization of the rectum and sigmoid
2. Endoscopy	_______	visualization from anus to cecum
3. Sigmoidoscopy	_______	visualization of esophagus, stomach, and small bowel
4. Barium swallow	_______	visualization of interior organs and structures using a fiberoptic instrument

Interactive Activity: With a partner, use the diagram to:

1. Identify the segments of the large intestine.
2. Follow the path of the colonoscopy procedure.
3. Identify the consistency of the stool as it moves through the intestinal tract (mushy, semi-liquid, and solid).

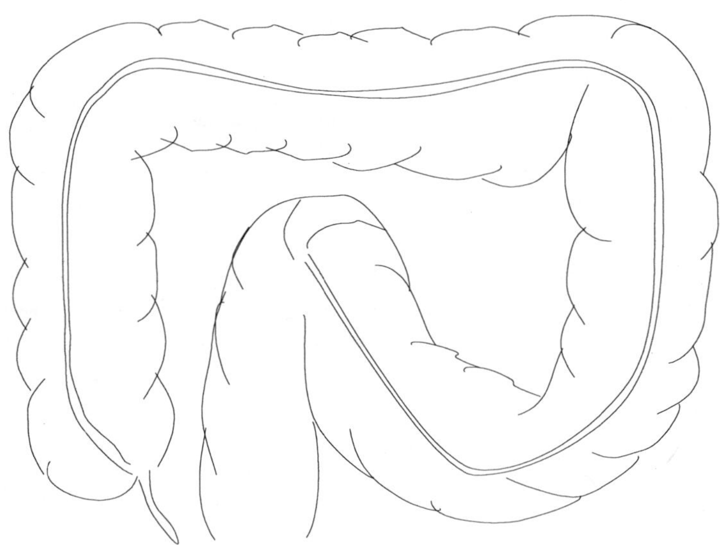

DIABETES MELLITUS

List the classic **signs and symptoms** of **diabetes mellitus**:

-
-
-

List other **signs** and **symptoms** associated with **hyperglycemia**:

-
-
-
-
-
-
-

Fill in the **circles** that identify the **signs and symptoms** associated with **hypoglycemia**.

- ○ Polyuria
- ○ Shakiness
- ○ Tremor
- ○ Glucosuria
- ○ Irritability
- ○ Confusion
- ○ Polydipsia
- ○ Dizziness
- ○ Blurred vision
- ○ Hunger
- ○ Slurred speech
- ○ Paresthesia
- ○ Tachycardia

Case Study: Marty, 20 years old, makes an appointment with her M.D. for complaints of feeling fatigued and lethargic for several days. She states that she has noticed that she has lost 15 lbs. She tells the M.D. that she does not understand why she has lost so much weight since she has been eating a lot. The M.D. inquires if she voids more than usual. Marty says that she does but that she thinks it is because of all the water that she is drinking all day.

Pertinent Terminology	Definition
Diabetes mellitus (DM)	
Type 1 diabetes mellitus	
Type 2 diabetes mellitus	
Insulin resistance	
Insulin	
Counter regulatory hormones	
Oral hypoglycemics agents	

The M.D. orders a fasting blood sugar (FBS) test and an FBS with a 2 hr post-prandial test for Marty. The following results are noted in Marty's clinic chart. **Write-in** the normal lab values for the test in the column provided.

Test	Results	Normal lab values
FBS	160 mg/dL	
2 hr PP	225 mg/dL	

Marty is informed that she has type 1 diabetes. **Fill in** the circle that correlates with the diagnosis and treatment of type 1.

- ❍ Oral hypoglycemics will be ordered
- ❍ Execise is part of the treatment plan
- ❍ Will need to monitor for S & S of hypoglycemia
- ❍ Insulin will be required everyday
- ❍ Will require blood sugar testing throughout the day
- ❍ Beta cells are producing insulin
- ❍ Will need to monitor for S & S of hyperglycemia
- ❍ Will not need insulin if follows diet

Interactive Activity: With a partner, use the **Key Points Box** and the **Follow-up case study** to **identify the response(s)** that should be included in responding to each question. **Write** the letter in the **Responses** section to identify the responses you have selected.

Key Points Box

A. "Usually ½ hr to 1 hr before breakfast"

B. "Insulin needs may change over time"

C. "Check blood sugar level"

D. "Always carry oral glucose tablets"

E. "Destroyed by the gastric enzymes"

F. "No"

G. "Drink orange, apple, or grape juice"

H. "Know the signs and symptoms of hypoglycemia"

Follow-up case study: Marty is started on Humulin NPH insulin 10 U q AM and NPH 5 U q PM. She is taught how to do self-monitoring blood glucose checks (SMBG) qid.

	Responses
1. "When is the best time to administer the AM insulin?"	______
2. "If I forget the pm dose of insulin, can I double the dose in the morning?"	______
3. "What should I do if I begin to get shaky and dizzy?"	______
4. "How do I prepare for a hypoglycemic reaction?"	______

COMPLICATIONS OF DIABETES MELLITUS

List the **causes** that precipitate **hypoglycemic episodes**:

» Incorrect dose
» alcohol
» ↑ phys. exercise
» drug interaction
» skip meal

For each line identify a specific **long term complication**, i.e., stroke, associated with Diabetes Mellitus.

Diabetes Mellitus

blindness
Atherosclerosis

List the **causes** that precipitate the development of **diabetic ketoacidosis**:

» incorrect insulin dose
» drug steroids
» stress illness

Case Study: Mr. Edwards, 56 years old, has been a diabetic for 25 years. He is admitted to the hospital for cerebral vascular accident. His wife says that her husband monitors his blood sugars daily and administers his own insulin. However, she tells the nurse that he does not always stick to his diet. She wonders whether this may have contributed to the CVA. Mr. Edwards has an order for NPH insulin 36 U q AM and NPH 17 U q PM with blood sugar fingersticks ac and hs and he is started on a sliding scale.

Pertinent Terminology	Definition
Lipoatrophy	depression in skin.
Lipohypertrophy	
Impaired glucose tolerance	
Somogyi effect	2 Am ↓ BG. 7 Am ↑ BG
Dawn phenomenon	3-4 Am ↑ BG
Diabetic ketoacidosis	due to hyperglycemia usu. Type I, ketones fr. decom fat. Require ↑ dose of insulin
Hyperglycemic Hyperosmolar Nonketotic coma	require ↓ dose of insulin.

Use the **case study, the follow-up information, and the nursing interventions below** to plan out Mr. Edward's morning care in the order of **priority**. Place a number, beginning with #1, in each box to indicate the sequence of the nursing care that should be delivered by the nurse.

Follow-up Information: The AM blood sugar fingerstick and insulin are to be done by the morning shift. Mr. Edwards is started on a diet containing thick liquids.

Nursing Interventions	Rationale
☐ Perform a body systems assessment	______
☐ Perform a fingerstick	______
☐ Take the AM vital signs	______
☐ Administer morning insulin	______
☐ Perform morning care	______
☐ Provide information regarding the complications of DM	______
☐ Assist with breakfast	______

Place a check (✔) next to the statements that are correct regarding the use of a sliding scale.

____ Only regular insulin is used

____ Dosage based on ac BS levels

____ May be combined with other insulins

____ Used for IDDM - Type 1 patients

____ Used for NIDDM - Type 2 patients

____ Used during periods of illness

Interactive Activity: The following nursing diagnosis is found on Mr. Edwards nursing care plan. With a partner, **write the 3 most important nursing interventions for the nursing diagnosis.**

Nursing Diagnosis	Nursing Interventions
Risk for Aspiration r/t impaired swallowing secondary to CVA	1. 2. 3

INSULIN THERAPY

List the **onset, peak, and duration** of the following insulins:

Short acting:

Onset ____________________

Peak ____________________

Duration ____________________

Intermediate acting:

Onset ____________________

Peak ____________________

Duration ____________________

Long acting:

Onset ____________________

Peak ____________________

Duration ____________________

Using the boxes on the left column write **(S)** if the insulin is Short acting, **(I)** if the insulin is intermediate acting and **(L)** if the insulin is long acting.

[ ]	Semilente	[ ]
[ ]	NPH	[ ]
[x]	Regular	[x]
[ ]	Ultralente	[ ]
[ ]	Lente	[ ]
[x]	Humulin R	[x]
[ ]	Humulin N	[ ]
[ ]	Humulog-Lispro	[x]

Place an **"X"** on the insulin(s) that may be given **IV** and that may be **mixed** with other

Case Study: Marty, 22 years old, has been on Humulin NPH insulin since her diagnosis of IDDM 2 years ago. Marty administers 12 U NPH with 5 U Regular insulin q AM and 4 U NPH q PM. She monitors her blood sugar qid ac and hs and routinely administers the AM insulin dose at 0700 and the PM dose at 1700. Marty maintains a daily chart of her blood sugar results.

Pertinent Terminology	Definition
Glucagon	
Glycogenolysis	breakdown conversion of glycogen to glucose in liver → glucagon.
Gluconeogenesis	
Glycosylated hemoglobin	shows long term overall
Glycosylated Albumin	
Oral Glucose Tolerance test	
Hypoglycemia	decrease in glucose level < 60. ✓ Pt. if symptomatic & asymptomatic.

From the case study, plot out Marty's morning dose of NPH and Regular insulin on the **Insulin Progression Graph**. Begin with the **onset (O)** followed by identifying the **peak of action (P)** of the insulin and the **duration (D)**.

Insulin Progression Graph
Onset → Peak → Duration

Length of time insulin remains in the body

	0700	0800	0900	1000	1100	1200	1300	1400	1500	1600	1700	1800	1900	2000	2100	2200	2300	2400	0100	0200	0300	0400	0500	0600
P																								
D																								
O																								

↑ AM NPH and Regular insulin administered

Marty eats a full breakfast at 0800 but is unable to eat lunch. Use the **Insulin Progression Graph** to indicate the time Marty would most likely experience a **hypoglycemic episode**? ________________

Select (✓) the most appropriate **snack** for Marty to eat **at this time**:

____ 6 saltine crackers
____ ½ chewy granola bar
____ 8 oz diet soda

Interactive Activity: With a partner, **underline** the **correct word** in each statement as it relates to the sentence and **provide a rationale** for your selection.

1. For the patient with IDDM, moderate exercise may have **hyperglycemic** or **hypoglycemic** effects.
   Rationale: ____

   ____

2. A patient with IDDM performs a fingerstick before exercising and the blood glucose results are 92 mg/dL. The patient should eat a snack **before** or **immediately after** exercising.
   Rationale: ____

   ____

3. Alcohol consumption causes **hypoglycemia** or **hyperglycemia** in the IDDM patient.
   Rationale: ____

   ____

LEGAL CONSIDERATIONS IN NURSING PRACTICE

List the **two types** of **torts**:

1. ______________________
2. ______________________

List the **four elements** that constitute **professional negligence**:

1. ______________________
2. ______________________
3. ______________________
4. ______________________

Draw a **line** to identify the **Unintentional Torts**

Fraud

Invasion of privacy

Unintentional Torts

Assault

Negligence

False Imprisonment

Libel

Malpractice

Case Study: Cassie, a new nursing student, is assigned to Mr. Watkins, a 73-yr.-old patient. Mr. Watkins has a kidney disease and has been in the hospital for 3 days. He is alert and wants to know everything about his treatment and questions the nurses all the time. The change of shift report indicates that he has had diarrhea all day. He keeps getting out of bed and the nurses feel that he is getting increasingly weak. Cassie is working with an experienced staff RN. The staff RN instructs Cassie to apply a vest restraint on Mr. Watkins if he gets up again to use the bathroom because she is concerned that he will fall and injure himself.

Pertinent Terminology	**Definition**
Assault	
Battery	
Libel	
Slander	
Negligence	
Malpractice	
Tort	
Informed consent	
Standard of care	

Use the information in the case study to **check-off** (✓) the statement or statements below that apply to the situation:

- ☐ A physician's order is not needed since Mr. Watkins is increasingly weak and the nurse has determined that he is a risk to himself.
- ☐ A thorough neurological assessment and documentation of unsafe behavior is important to document prior to applying a restraint. An order is necessary.
- ☐ Application of a vest restraint against Mr. Watkins wishes may be considered assault and battery and may have legal implications.
- ☐ It is important to follow the instructions of the experienced RN since she alone is responsible for the care that Mr. Watkins receives.

Interactive Activity: With a partner, use the case studies below to, **(1)** check-off (✓) the most appropriate action(s) and **(2)** answer the question at the end of the case study.

Case Study	Action(s)
Cindi, a second year nursing student, has been under a lot of personal stress. She tells another student that she gave her patient the wrong amount of sedative in the morning, but that she took no action because the patient was fine and she checked his vital signs all day. Cindi is an excellent student and will not allow this to happen again.	☐ The patient was fine—take no action ☐ Fill out an Incident Report ☐ The instructor should be notified ☐ The charge nurse should be notified

Cindi **has** **or** **has not** **been negligent, because** ______________________________
Circle one

____

Mark is a graduate nurse and started working as soon as he received his RN license. He administered medications one evening to a patient with a nasogastric tube. After administering the medication, the patient began coughing and Mark noticed the nasogastric tube was significantly out of the patient's nose.	☐ Notify the M.D. ☐ Reinsert the tube & listen for placement ☐ Fill out an Incident Report ☐ Readminister the medications

Mark **has** **or** **has not** **been negligent, because** ______________________________
Circle one

____

SECTION TWO

Priority-Setting and Decision-Making Activities

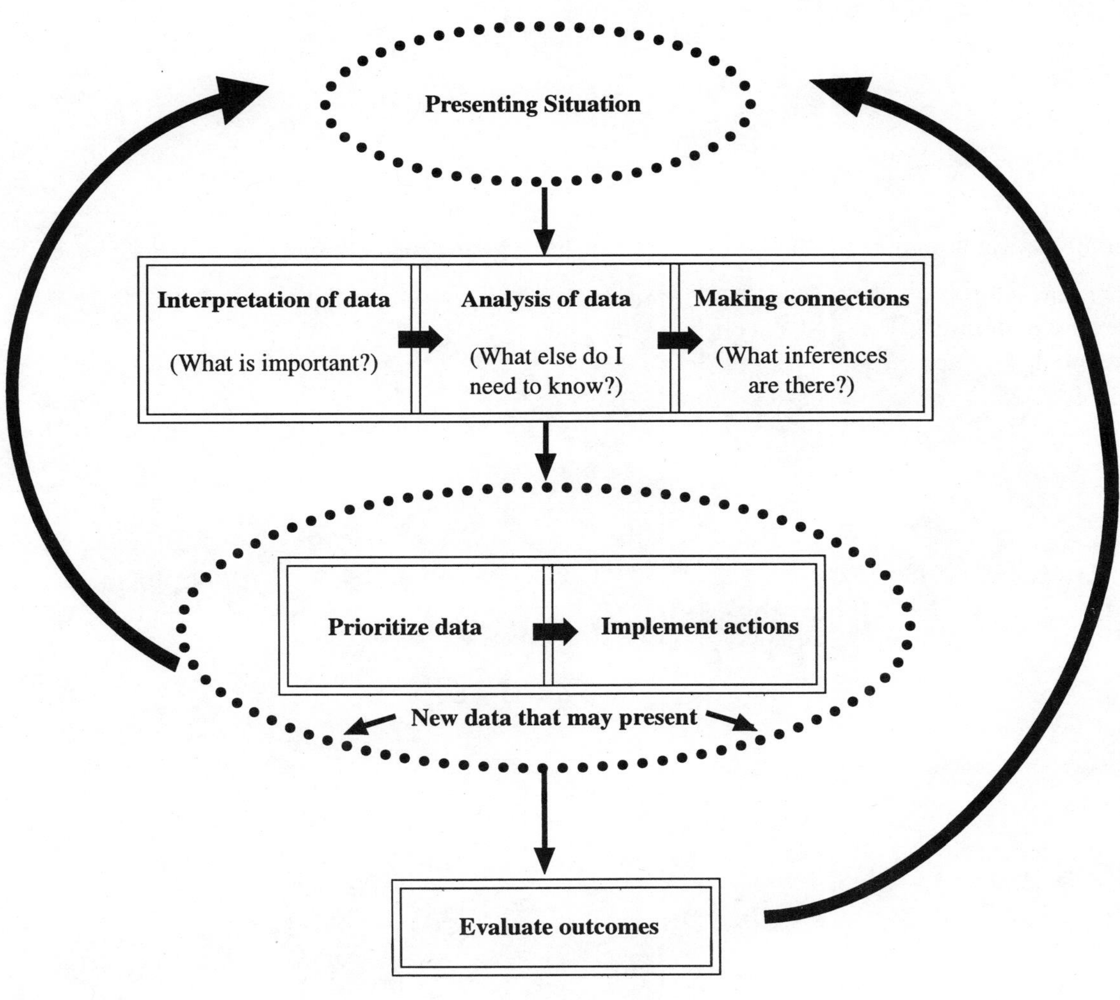

THE PATIENT UNDERGOING SURGERY

Mr. Hatori, age 60, was admitted with persistent abdominal pain. He states he has had nausea and vomiting and has noticed a 10 lb weight loss within the last 2 months. He is diagnosed with gastric cancer and is scheduled for a subtotal gastrectomy in the morning. He has Demerol 75 mg with Phenergan 25 mg IM q3-4 hr prn pain and Mylanta 30 cc p.o. q2h prn abdominal pain. Mr. Hatori is very anxious after speaking with his physician and refuses to sign the surgical consent. He tells the nurse that he is having abdominal pain and "wants his pain shot right now." The nurse notes that it is just about three hours since his last pain medication.

Instructions: Prioritize the following **nursing interventions** as you, the nurse, would do them to initially take care of Mr. Hatori. Write a number in the box to identify the order of your interventions (**#1** = first intervention, **#2** = second intervention, etc.) and state a **rationale** for each intervention.

INTERVENTIONS	PRIORITY #	RATIONALE
◇ Administer IM pain med.	☐	______
◇ Sit and talk with patient	☐	______
◇ Give Mylanta 30 cc	☐	______
◇ Offer to call a family member	☐	______
◇ Notify physician	☐	______

KEY POINTS TO CONSIDER: ______

______

______

Mr. Hatori does consent to have surgery and returns to the medical unit postoperative. He has an IV of Lactated Ringer's infusing at 125 cc/hr and you note the following:

1) P. 90 - R. 20 - BP 130/76
2) He is alert, oriented, skin warm and dry
3) N/G tube draining brown-reddish drainage (300 cc in the last 4 hours)
4) Indwelling urinary catheter draining light yellow urine (700 cc in the last 4 hours)

✓✓✓ **Interactive Activity:** With a partner, **do the following: (1) based on the current assessment, select** the **one nursing diagnosis** that is of priority at this time, **(2) provide a rationale** for your selection, and **(3) list three nursing interventions** that meet the needs of Mr. Hatori:

All of the following Nursing Diagnoses may apply to Mr. Hatori.

Risk for infection, Pain, Anxiety, Ineffective airway clearance, Fatigue, Impaired physical mobility, Altered nutrition: Less than body requirements, Knowledge deficit, Risk for fluid volume deficit, Fear.

Nursing Diagnosis	Rationale	Nursing Interventions
		1. 2. 3.

✓✓✓ Several hours after surgery you note that Mr. Hatori is very restless and you assess:

R. 32 - P. 130 - BP 108/70, N/G drainage 200 cc bright red drainage, skin cool, c/o pain

Instructions: Based on the situation above, identify and write the **priority problem** in the box below. Then, starting with the small box labeled **#1 prioritize** the **nursing interventions** for this situation and **identify** your plan for follow-up care for Mr. Hatori.

NURSING INTERVENTIONS

A. Monitor P, R, BP

B. Document assessment/nursing care

C. Prepare for gastric lavage

D. Plan to start oxygen therapy

E. Stay with Mr. Hatori

F. Notify physician

DECISION-MAKING DIAGRAM

New Action Plan

#1 #2 #3 #4 #5 #6

Priority Problem

NOTES

THE PATIENT WITH AN INTESTINAL OBSTRUCTION

Mrs. Wooley, 56 yrs. old, is hospitalized with the diagnosis of small bowel obstruction. She has an N/G tube to low continuous suction, draining dark brown drainage and an IV of D5/0.45% NS with 30 mEq KCl infusing at 100 cc/hr. Her skin is warm, dry and her mucous membranes are dry. Her abdomen is distended with hyperactive bowel sounds in the right upper and lower quadrants. The nursing assistant reports that Mrs. Wooley just vomited 100 cc dark brown secretions.

Instructions: Prioritize the following **nursing interventions** as you would do them to initially take care of Mrs. Wooley. Write a number in the box to identify the order of your interventions (**#1** = first intervention, **#2** = second intervention, etc.) and state a **rationale** for each intervention.

INTERVENTIONS	PRIORITY #	RATIONALE
◊ Provide thorough mouth care	☐	______
◊ Assess abdomen, measure abdominal girth	☐	______
◊ Assess N/G tube and suction	☐	______
◊ Take the vital signs	☐	______
◊ Ensure Mrs. Wooley is in semi-Fowler's position	☐	______

KEY POINTS TO CONSIDER: ______

After 48 hours Mrs. Wooley's abdomen is less distended and the current assessment findings include:

1) Hgb 9.2 g, Hct 29%, K^+ 3.1 mEq, Na^+ 145 mEq
2) T. 98.8, P. 92 - irregular, R. 20, BP 152/94
3) N/G tube draining dark brown drainage (250 cc in the last 8 hours)
4) Pain on a 1-10 scale = 4
5) No stool or passing of flatus, urine output last 24 hrs 700 cc

✓✓✓ **Interactive Activity:** With a partner, **do the following: (1) based on the current assessment, select** the **one nursing diagnosis** that is of priority at this time, **(2) provide a rationale** for your selection, and **(3) list three nursing interventions** that meet the needs of Mrs. Wooley.

All of the following Nursing Diagnoses may apply to Mrs. Wooley.

Risk for infection, Pain, Anxiety, Ineffective airway clearance, Altered nutrition: Less than body requirements, Knowledge deficit, Fluid volume deficit, Risk for impaired skin integrity, Fear, Sleep pattern disturbance.

Nursing Diagnosis	Rationale	Nursing Interventions
		1. 2. 3.

✓✓✓ The next day, Mrs. Wooley's assessment included the following: N/G output 500 cc and urine output 100 cc dark amber during the night shift. Faint bowel sounds, capillary refill >5 secs. Weak, lethargic, and disoriented. Mucous membranes dry. Orthostatic BP 148/90 (lying); 124/84 (standing)

Instructions: Based on the situation above, identify and write the **priority problem** in the box below. Then, starting with the small box labeled **#1 prioritize** the **nursing interventions** for this situation and **identify** your follow-up action plan for Mrs. Wooley.

NURSING INTERVENTIONS

A. Monitor IV fluid replacement

B. Inform RN/physician

C. Orient Mrs. Wooley

D. Provide oral care

E. Raise side rails

F. Take vital signs

DECISION-MAKING DIAGRAM

New Action Plan

#1 #2 #3 #4 #5 #6

Priority Problem

NOTES____________________

THE PATIENT WITH A COLOSTOMY

Mrs. Potts, 42 yrs. old, had surgery today for colon cancer. She was transferred to her room two hours ago. In the taped evening shift tape report you learn that she has a sigmoid colostomy with a colostomy bag in place, a clean dry surgical dressing, an N/G tube to low continuous wall suction draining dark brown drainage, a right central line with TPN infusing at 83 cc/hr, and an IV of D5/NS with a PCA (morphine sulfate) set to deliver 1 mg/6 min per patient demand.

Instructions: Prioritize the following **nursing interventions** as you, the nurse, would do them to initially take care of Mrs. Potts. Write a number in the box to identify the order of your interventions (**#1** = first intervention, **#2** = second intervention, etc.) and state a **rationale** for each intervention.

INTERVENTIONS	PRIORITY #	RATIONALE
◇ Assess surgical dressing and stoma	☐	__________
◇ Take the vital signs	☐	__________
◇ Assess pain level	☐	__________
◇ Check N/G tube and drainage	☐	__________
◇ Check IV site, TPN and PCA setting	☐	__________

KEY POINTS TO CONSIDER: ____________________

The **first postop day** assessment was significant for the following signs and symptoms:

1) Bowel sounds absent
2) Mrs. Potts moans when she turns in bed
3) Has a weak, ineffective cough
4) Stoma swollen and reddened

✓✓✓ **Interactive Activity:** With a partner, **do the following: (1) select** the **one nursing diagnosis** that is of priority at this time, **(2) provide a rationale** for your selection, and **(3) list three nursing interventions** that assist to meet the needs of the patient:

All of the following Nursing Diagnoses may apply to Mrs. Potts.

Risk for infection, Risk for impaired skin integrity, Pain, Anxiety, Ineffective airway clearance, Fatigue, Impaired physical mobility, Altered nutrition: Less than body requirements, Body image disturbance, Risk for fluid volume deficit, Fear.

Nursing Diagnosis	Rationale	Nursing Interventions
		1. 2. 3.

✓✓✓ On the morning of the **third postop day**, the N/G tube was removed per physician order and Mrs. Potts was started on a clear liquid diet. In the afternoon the assessment findings included:

Stoma edematous and pale, abdomen distended, c/o of pain.

Instructions: Based on the **third postop day** assessment, identify and write the **priority problem** in the box below. Then, starting with the small box labeled **#1, prioritize** the **nursing interventions** listed and **identify** your action plan for the follow-up care of Mrs. Potts.

NURSING INTERVENTIONS

A. Take the vital signs

B. Prepare to insert N/G tube

C. Assess colostomy bag and stoma

D. Notify physician stat

E. Place on NPO

F. Check IV patency

DECISION-MAKING DIAGRAM

New Action Plan

#1 #2 #3 #4 #5 #6

Priority Problem

NOTES

THE PATIENT WITH COLON CANCER

Mr. Sweetwater, 65 yrs. old, has colon cancer. He is admitted for a colon resection. His current medical history is significant for complaints of changes in bowel habits—constipation, passing of bloody stools, abdominal pain, and weight loss. His past medical condition includes history of coronary artery disease and hypertension. In addition to antihypertensive medication, he takes Aspirin 81 mg p.o. qd. In preparation for surgery, his current orders include NPO, insert an N/G tube, and a saline lock. His 6:00 AM vital signs are T. 98 - P. 78 - R. 20 - BP 162/90. He is to receive his preop medication at 12:00 PM today. The nurse gets out of report at 8:00 AM.

Instructions: Prioritize the five **nursing interventions** as you, the nurse, would do them to initially take care of Mr. Sweetwater. Write a number in the box to identify the order of your interventions (#1 = first intervention, #2 = second intervention, etc.) and state a **rationale** for each intervention.

INTERVENTIONS	PRIORITY #	RATIONALE
◊ Perform a body systems assessment	☐	
◊ Take the vital signs	☐	
◊ Insert saline lock	☐	
◊ Insert N/G tube	☐	
◊ Check surgical consent	☐	

KEY POINTS TO CONSIDER:

A colon resection is done on Mr. Sweetwater. The **first postop day** assessment includes:

1) Lactated Ringer's infusing at 100 cc/hr and PCA with morphine sulfate
2) Elastic stockings. Intermittent compression device for 24 hrs
3) N/G tube to low continuous suction draining brown-greenish fluid
4) Wants to stay in a low Fowler's position
5) Short and shallow respirations

✓✓✓ **Interactive Activity:** With a partner, **do the following: (1)** based on the **first post-operative day assessment, select** the **one nursing diagnosis** that is of priority at this time, **(2) provide a rationale** for your selection, and **(3) list three nursing interventions** that meet the needs of Mr. Sweetwater:

All of the following Nursing Diagnoses may apply to Mr. Sweetwater.

Risk for infection, Pain, Anxiety, Ineffective airway clearance, Altered nutrition: Less than body requirements, Knowledge deficit, Risk for fluid volume deficit, Risk for impaired skin integrity, Risk for altered tissue perfusion, Fear.

Nursing Diagnosis	Rationale	Nursing Interventions
		1. 2. 3.

✓✓✓ On the **fourth postop** day you assess the following signs and symptoms on Mr. Sweetwater:

c/o tenderness in the right calf with a positive Homan's sign, 2+ right ankle/calf edema, right calf warmer to touch than left calf.

Instructions: Based on the **fourth postop** assessment, identify and write the **priority problem** in the box below. Then, starting with the small box labeled **#1 prioritize** the **nursing interventions** for this situation and **identify** your plan for follow-up care for Mr. Sweetwater.

NURSING INTERVENTIONS

A. Elevate right extremity

B. Notify physician

C. Maintain bedrest

D. Allay Mr. Sweetwater's concerns

E. Administer mild analgesic if ordered

F. Assess pedal pulses

DECISION-MAKING DIAGRAM

New Action Plan

#1 #2 #3 #4 #5 #6

Priority Problem

NOTES

THE PATIENT WITH TPN

You are assigned to care for Mrs. Fox. In report you learn that her diarrhea is decreasing and her current VS are 98.8 - 76 - 18 BP 130/84. She has complained of pain in her right leg.

VS q4hrs I & O (✔) Weigh qd BRP with assist prn	Right central line inserted 3/16 TPN @ 83 cc/hr per pump Lipids 10% (M-W-F) BS Fingersticks q6hrs (6-12-6-12)	Diet: NPO Routine med: Vit. K 10 mg SC q Mon
Admit date: 3/16 Name: Fox, Jane M. Age: 55	Dx: Dehydration/Diarrhea Hx of Crohn's-acute exacerbation Atrial fibrillation	Reg, Ins. 2 U if BS = 180 - 200 mg Call M.D. if BS >200 mg

Instructions: Prioritize the five **nursing interventions** as you would do them to take care of Mrs. Fox. Write a number in the box to identify the order of your interventions (**#1** = first intervention, **#2** = second intervention, etc.) and state a **rationale** for each intervention.

INTERVENTIONS **PRIORITY #** **RATIONALE**

◇ Perform a body systems physical assessment

◇ Assess Homan's sign

◇ Assess central line for patency and central line dressing

◇ Get 0600 blood sugar results

◇ Assess for right arm edema and neck vein distention

KEY POINTS TO CONSIDER:

Mrs. Fox was taken to x-ray an hour ago. Upon her return to the unit, the IV pump is beeping and you are informed that the machine has been beeping for a long time. You assess the following:

1) TPN not infusing
2) Skin warm, diaphoretic, c/o nervousness and rapid heartbeat
3) VS 98-118- 26 BP 136/80

✓✓✓ **Interactive Activity:** With a partner, **do the following: (1) select** the **one nursing diagnosis** that is of priority at this time, **(2) provide a rationale** for your selection, and **(3) list the nursing interventions** that assist to meet the needs of the patient:

All of the following Nursing Diagnoses may apply to Mrs. Fox.

Anxiety, Risk for infection, Risk for activity intolerance, Risk for fluid volume excess, Impaired tissue integrity, Risk for altered tissue perfusion, Altered nutrition: Less than body requirements, Risk for injury: hypoglycemia, Knowledge deficit.

Nursing Diagnosis	Rationale	Nursing Interventions
		1. 2. 3.

✓✓✓ **Three hours later,** Mrs. Fox's family calls the nursing station to say that Mrs. Fox is having difficulty breathing. You go into Mrs. Fox's room and assess the following:

c/o chest pain, R. 36, P. 110, coughing, dyspnea, anxiousness

Instructions: Based on the **three hours later** situation, identify and write the **priority problem** in the box below. Then, starting with the small box labeled **#1 prioritize** the **nursing interventions** for this situation and **identify** your follow-up action plan for Mrs. Fox.

NURSING INTERVENTIONS

A. Stay with Mrs. Fox

B. Raise HOB

C. Take P - R - BP

D. Monitor O_2 saturation level

E. Notify RN/M.D.

F. Administer oxygen

DECISION-MAKING DIAGRAM

New Action Plan

#1 #2 #3 #4 #5 #6

Priority Problem

NOTES____________________

THE PATIENT WITH CIRRHOSIS OF THE LIVER

Mr. Saul Uribe, 46 yrs. old, was admitted with the diagnosis of Laënnec's cirrhosis. In the evening report you learn that he is jaundiced, has ascites, and is experiencing increasing SOB. His VS at 12:00 p.m. were 99-94-34 and 140/90. The vital signs are consistent with previous recordings. You get out of report at 4:30 p.m. The nursing care Kardex includes the following orders:

VS q4hrs I & O (✔) Neuro cks q4hrs	Saline lock (✔)	Diet: ↑ CHO, 30 g Prot., 2 g Na^+
CBC, serum ammonia } today AST, ALT, PT	Bedrest with BRP	Routine med: Amphogel 30 cc po qid Furosemide 40 mg IV qd Aldactone 50 mg po bid
Procedure: Abd. Paracentesis at 5:00 pm today	Weigh daily Measure abd. girth daily	

Instructions: Prioritize the five **nursing interventions** as you would do them to take care of Mr. Uribe. Write a number in the box to identify the order of your interventions (**#1** = first intervention, **#2** = second intervention, etc.) and state a **rationale** for each intervention.

INTERVENTIONS	PRIORITY #	RATIONALE
◇ Ensure consent form is signed	☐	______
◇ Take the vital signs	☐	______
◇ Perform a body systems physical assessment	☐	______
◇ Ensure abdominal paracentesis equipment is on the unit	☐	______
◇ Have Mr. Uribe void	☐	______

KEY POINTS TO CONSIDER: ______

The physician performs the abdominal paracentesis on Mr. Uribe and removes 2.5 L of fluid. VS during the procedure were pulse 90, resp. 32, BP 136/86. Post procedure you assess:

1) VS: P. 94, R. 24 BP 136/86
2) Dressing at the abdominal puncture site clean
3) Mr. Uribe is lying in a semi-Fowler's position
4) He is alert and oriented, although slow to respond

✓✓✓ **Interactive Activity:** With a partner, **do the following: (1) select** the **one nursing diagnosis** that is of priority at this time, **(2) provide a rationale** for your selection, and **(3) list the nursing interventions** that assist to meet the needs of the patient.

All of the following Nursing Diagnoses may apply to Mr. Uribe.

Risk for injury: Fall, Risk for infection, Impaired skin integrity, Risk for impaired physical mobility, Pain, Altered nutrition: Less than body requirements, Risk for altered thought processes, Risk for activity intolerance, Impaired tissue integrity, Fluid volume excess, Risk for fluid volume deficit, Ineffective breathing pattern, Body image disturbance, Sleep pattern disturbance, Fatigue, Altered comfort.

Nursing Diagnosis	Rationale	Nursing Interventions
		1. 2. 3. 4.

✓✓✓ The **lab results for** today are:

PT 40 secs.	Serum ammonia 70 μg/dL	Hgb 10.6 g/dL	Hct 30%
WBC 3500/mm^3	Platelets 100,000/mm^3	AST 100 U/L	ALT 500 U/L

Instructions: Based on the **lab results** data, identify and write the **priority problem** in the box below. Then, starting with the small box labeled **#1 prioritize** the **nursing interventions** for this situation and **identify** your follow-up action plan for Mr. Uribe.

NURSING INTERVENTIONS

A. Monitor the VS

B. Assess for petechiae

C. Check stool for occult blood

D. Monitor urine color

E. Check neuro status

F. Notify RN/M.D.

Priority Problem

DECISION-MAKING DIAGRAM

New Action Plan

#1 #2 #3 #4 #5 #6

NOTES

THE PATIENT WITH HEPATIC ENCEPHALOPATHY

Mr. Uribe, 47 yrs. old, is admitted with the diagnosis of hepatic encephalopathy related to his advanced liver cirrhosis. The night report indicates that he was awake most of the night and very restless most of shift. The nursing care kardex has the following orders:

VS q4hrs I & O (✔) Neuro cks q4hrs Serum ammonia, K^+ today Code Status: No code	D5W at 100 cc/hr #20 g RFA - inserted today Bedrest with BRP Weigh daily	Diet: ↑ CHO, 50 g Prot., 4g Na^+ Routine med: Neomycin 1 g po q6h Lactulose 30 cc bid

As you enter his room you notice that Mr. Uribe is sleeping.

Instructions: Prioritize the five **nursing interventions** as you would do them to take care of Mr. Uribe. Write a number in the box to identify the order of your interventions (**#1** = first intervention, **#2** = second intervention, etc.) and state a **rationale** for each intervention.

INTERVENTIONS	PRIORITY #	RATIONALE
◇ Take the vital signs	☐	______
◇ Assess the LOC and orientation	☐	______
◇ Check current serum ammonia and K^+ levels	☐	______
◇ Perform a body systems physical assessment	☐	______
◇ Assist Mr. Uribe with ADLs	☐	______

KEY POINTS TO CONSIDER: ______

______

______

Mr. Uribe has refused his morning dose of lactulose and you further assess:

1) He refused the lactulose the previous day
2) No BM for 2 days
3) Irritable, speech slurred
4) Responds slowly to verbal communication

✓✓✓ **Interactive Activity:** With a partner, **do the following: (1) select** the **one nursing diagnosis** that is of priority at this time, **(2) provide a rationale** for your selection, and **(3) list the nursing interventions** that assist to meet the needs of the patient.

All of the following Nursing Diagnoses may apply to Mr. Uribe.

Risk for injury: falls, Risk for infection, Impaired skin integrity, Self-care deficit: bathing/hygiene, Risk for impaired physical mobility, Risk for Constipation, Altered nutrition: Less than body requirements, Activity intolerance, Impaired tissue integrity, Fluid volume excess, Ineffective breathing pattern, Fatigue, Altered thought processes, Sleep pattern disturbance, Altered comfort.

Nursing Diagnosis	Rationale	Nursing Interventions
		1. 2. 3. 4.

✓✓✓ You return from lunch at **1:00 PM** and you are informed of the following:

Mr. Uribe is becoming increasingly confused and lethargic. He did not eat lunch.

Instructions: Based on the **1:00 PM** information, identify and write the **priority problem** in the box below. Then, starting with the small box labeled **#1 prioritize** the **nursing interventions** for this situation and **identify** your follow-up action plan for Mr. Uribe.

NURSING INTERVENTIONS

A. Inform RN/physician

B. Document assessment findings

C. Take the vital signs

D. Notify the relatives

E. Stay with patient

F. Raise the bedrails

DECISION-MAKING DIAGRAM

New Action Plan

#1 #2 #3 #4 #5 #6

Priority Problem

NOTES____________________

THE PATIENT WITH DIABETES MELLITUS

The nurse is assigned to a 56-year-old Hispanic female, Mrs. Garcia, admitted with the Dx. of End Stage Renal Disease. She has a thirty year history of Type 1 DM. She is scheduled to have hemodialysis this AM. The night nurse indicates that she has a 2 cm dry ulcerated circular area on the lateral outer aspect of her right great toe and an AV fistula in the right forearm. She has an order for NPH Insulin 15 U SC q AM and bloodsugar fingerstick qid. It is 0730 when the nurse gets out of report and breakfast arrives on the unit at 0800.

Instructions: Prioritize the five **nursing interventions** as you would do them to take care of Mrs. Garcia. Write a number in the box to identify the order of your interventions (**#1** = first intervention, **#2** = second intervention, etc.) and state a **rationale** for each intervention.

INTERVENTIONS	PRIORITY #	RATIONALE
◇ Check chart for blood sugar fingerstick results	1	
◇ Assess AV fistula	4	
◇ Administer NPH 15 U SC	2	
◇ Get patient ready for breakfast	5	
◇ Perform a body systems physical assessment	3	

KEY POINTS TO CONSIDER:

Mrs. Garcia is still waiting for her dialysis treatment. At 1000 the M.D. leaves the following orders:

Sliding scale - for fingerstick blood sugar: 225 - 250 give 10 U Reg Ins.
200 - 224 give 5 U Reg Ins.
150 - 199 give 2 U Reg Ins.
< 150 no insulin

You do a fingerstick at 1130. The results are 236. You will give ___10 U___ Regular Insulin.

✓✓✓ **Interactive Activity:** With a partner, **do the following: (1) select** the **one nursing diagnosis** that is of priority at this time, **(2) provide a rationale** for your selection, and **(3) list nursing interventions** that assist to meet the needs of the patient:

All of the following Nursing Diagnoses may apply to Mrs. Garcia.

Risk for infection, Risk for impaired skin integrity, Impaired physical mobility, Altered patterns of elimination, Altered sexual pattern, Sensory/perceptual alterations, Fatigue, Fluid volume excess, Fluid volume deficit, Altered nutrition: Less than body requirements

Nursing Diagnosis	Rationale	Nursing Interventions
Fluid Vol excess pt. cannot get rid of waste urine.		1. 2. 3. 4.

✓✓✓ As you take her 1300 VS you note the following signs and symptoms:
Irritability, skin warm, moist, VS - 36.8 - 100 - 18, BP 150/84. She is c/o dizziness and "feeling funny." hypoglycemia.

Instructions: Based on the situation above, identify and write the **priority problem** in the box below. Then, starting with the small box labeled **#1 prioritize** the **nursing interventions** for this situation and **identify** your plan for follow-up care for Mrs. Garcia.

NURSING INTERVENTIONS **DECISION-MAKING DIAGRAM**

A. Document findings/nursing care
B. Retake fingerstick bloodsugar stat
C. Check fingerstick bloodsugar in 15 min
D. Give 4 ozs apple juice
E. Report findings stat to an RN
F. Raise the side rails

New Action Plan

#1	#2	#3	#4	#5	#6
E	F	B.	D	C	A

Priority Problem

NOTES

THE PATIENT UNDERGOING HEMODIALYSIS

Ms. Gladys Abbott, 52 yrs. old, has ESRD and has just been started on dialysis. She has an AV fistula in the right forearm and is scheduled for dialysis at 0800 today. The night nurse reports that the fistula has a good thrill and bruit. Ms. Abbott's BP is 160/102. You leave the report room at 0730 after noting the following orders from the nursing care kardex:

VS q8hrs I & O (✔) Weigh daily H & H, serum ferritin (✔) Serum iron saturation (✔)	IV: Saline lock—left hand Routine medications: Vasotec 10 mg po qd 0800 Folic acid 1 mg po qd 0800 $FeSo_4$ 325 po tid c̄ meals Epogen 300 u SC M-W-F	Diet: 70 g Protein, 2g Na^+, 2g K^+ Fluid restriction 1000 cc/day

Instructions: Prioritize the five **nursing interventions** as you would do them to take care of Ms. Abbott. Write a number in the box to identify the order of your interventions (**#1** = first intervention, **#2** = second intervention, etc.) and state a **rationale** for each intervention.

INTERVENTIONS	PRIORITY #	RATIONALE
◇ Take the VS (BP on the left arm)	☐	______
◇ Perform body systems physical assessment	☐	______
◇ Weigh patient/ensure Ms. Abbott has been weighed	☐	______
◇ Assess AV fistula for thrill & bruit	☐	______
◇ Hold folic acid and Vasotec	☐	______

KEY POINTS TO CONSIDER: ______

Ordered lab studies were drawn prior to dialysis. The results of the morning lab are:

1) Hgb 9.5 g/dL, Hct 28%
2) Ferritin 60 ng/L
3) Serum iron saturation 18%
4) K^+ 5.0 mEq

✓✓✓ **Interactive Activity:** With a partner, **do the following: (1) select** the **one nursing diagnosis** that is of priority at this time, **(2) provide a rationale** for your selection, and **(3) list the nursing interventions** that assist to meet the needs of the patient.

All of the following Nursing Diagnoses may apply to Ms. Abbott.

Risk for injury, Knowledge deficit, Fear, Anxiety, Risk for infection, Impaired tissue integrity, Risk for Alteration in sensory/perceptual, Constipation, Fluid volume excess, Fluid volume deficit, Body image disturbance, Risk for impaired physical mobility, Altered tissue perfusion, Altered nutrition: Less than body requirements, Fatigue.

Nursing Diagnosis	Rationale	Nursing Interventions
		1. 2. 3. 4.

✓✓✓ **After the dialysis treatment,** Ms. Abbott is restless and you assess:

c/o headache, pruritus, nausea, change in LOC, twitching, confusion

Instructions: Based on **after the dialysis treatment** data, identify and write the **priority problem** in the box below. Then, starting with the small box labeled **#1 prioritize** the **nursing interventions** for this situation and **identify** your follow-up action plan for Ms. Abbott.

NURSING INTERVENTIONS

A. Take the VS

B. Notify RN/physician

C. Maintain calm, quiet environment

D. Stay with patient

E. Monitor neuro status

F. Document assessment findings

DECISION-MAKING DIAGRAM

New Action Plan

#1 #2 #3 #4 #5 #6

Priority Problem

NOTES

THE PATIENT WITH PERIPHERAL ARTERIAL DISEASE

Mr. Ed Lin, 70 yrs. old, is sent to the hospital after visiting his physician with c/o increasing painful muscle cramps after ambulating. He lives alone and his medical history is significant for hypertension.

The nursing care kardex has the following admit orders:

VS q4hrs I & O (✔) Pedal pulse check q4hrs Bedrest with BRP CBC Ed Lin Age: 70	Insert Saline lock Drsg chgs: Clean ulcerated area on left foot with Betadine - apply dry sterile 4x4s Dx. Peripheral Arterial Disease	Diet: Mech Soft Routine med: Trental 400 mg po tid Dipyridamole 50 mg po tid

You are assigned to begin his admission. You note that he is alert, but hard of hearing. He has a bandage around his left foot. He tells you he uses this to keep his shoe from rubbing his foot.

Instructions: Prioritize the five **nursing interventions** as you would do them to take care of Mr. Lin. Write a number in the box to identify the order of your interventions (**#1** = first intervention, **#2** = second intervention, etc.) and state a **rationale** for each intervention.

INTERVENTIONS	PRIORITY #	RATIONALE
◇ Take the vital signs	☐	______
◇ Assess bilateral pedal pulses	☐	______
◇ Orient to hospital room	☐	______
◇ Perform a body systems physical assessment	☐	______
◇ Apply sterile dressing to left foot	☐	______

KEY POINTS TO CONSIDER:______

______

______

You assist Mr. Lin to the bathroom, upon his return to bed you note the following:

1) Bilateral lower extremities—reddish blue in color
2) Bilateral pedal pulses weak (1+), capillary refill > 3 sec.
3) Lower extremities cool to touch
4) Gait slow, needs assistance

✓✓✓ **Interactive Activity:** With a partner, **do the following: (1) select** the **one nursing diagnosis** that is of priority at this time, **(2) provide a rationale** for your selection, and **(3) list the nursing interventions** that assist to meet the needs of the patient.

All of the following Nursing Diagnoses may apply to Mr. Lin.

Risk for injury: fall, Knowledge deficit, Risk for infection, Impaired skin integrity, Self-care deficit, Risk for impaired physical mobility, Altered peripheral tissue perfusion, Activity intolerance, Impaired tissue integrity, Pain.

Nursing Diagnosis	Rationale	Nursing Interventions
		1. 2. 3. 4.

✓✓✓ You **remove the bandage** from the left foot and you note:

A circular ulcerated area with two toes blackened and shriveled

Instructions: Based on **removal of the bandage** information, identify and write the **priority problem** in the box below. Then, starting with the small box labeled **#1 prioritize** the **nursing interventions** for this situation and **identify** your follow-up action plan for Mr. Lin.

NURSING INTERVENTIONS

A. Inform RN/physician

B. Measure ulcerated area

C. Put sterile gloves on

D. Cleanse area with Betadine

E. Apply sterile dressings

F. Document assessment findings

DECISION-MAKING DIAGRAM

New Action Plan

#1 #2 #3 #4 #5 #6

Priority Problem

NOTES

THE PATIENT WITH CHEST PAIN

Mrs. Tracey, 56 yrs. old, was admitted after experiencing chest pain. She has coronary artery disease and smokes 1 pack of cigarettes a day. Her father died of heart disease and she has a brother with hypertension. Her VS are 98-90-26, BP 164/100. Mrs. Tracey has been taking verapamil, Procardia, and Tenormin. Mrs. Tracey will continue with her usual cardiac and blood pressure medications and is also started on baby aspirin, Colace, and Lovastatin. Nitroglycerin tabs. 0.4 mg SL are ordered prn chest pain and Mylanta 30 cc q2h prn. She has BRP with assistance, a saline lock, and oxygen at 2-3 L/NC to keep O_2 sat $>96\%$. The night nurse reports that Mrs. Tracey is upset about not being able to smoke. Mrs. Tracey is requesting to use the commode as you start your shift.

Instructions: Prioritize the five **nursing interventions** as you would do them to initially take care of Mrs. Tracey. Write a number in the box to identify the order of your interventions (**#1** = first intervention, **#2** = second intervention, etc.) and state a **rationale** for each intervention.

INTERVENTIONS	PRIORITY #	RATIONALE
◇ Take the vital signs	☐	______
◇ Assist to commode	☐	______
◇ Perform a body systems physical assessment	☐	______
◇ Check O_2 saturation level	☐	______
◇ Talk with Mrs. Tracey	☐	______

KEY POINTS TO CONSIDER: ______

After breakfast Mrs. Tracey continues to be upset. She states that she is constipated and above all wants to smoke. She is getting increasingly upset. You observe the following:

1) Abdomen round, bowel sounds present in all four quadrants
2) Breakfast intake 30%
3) LBM 2 days ago
4) O_2 saturation level 93%

✓✓✓ **Interactive Activity:** With a partner, **do the following: (1) select** the **one nursing diagnosis** that is of priority at this time, **(2) provide a rationale** for your selection, and **(3) list the nursing interventions** that assist to meet the needs of the patient:

All of the following Nursing Diagnoses may apply to Mrs. Tracey.

Pain, Knowledge deficit, Anxiety, Risk for noncompliance, Risk for decreased cardiac output, Activity intolerance, Altered tissue perfusion:cardiopulmonary, Risk for impaired skin integrity, Constipation, Altered health maintenance.

Nursing Diagnosis	Rationale	Nursing Interventions
		1. 2. 3. 4.

✓✓✓ At **10:00 AM** the nursing assistant reports that Mrs. Tracey is experiencing chest pain. You assess and note that she has cool, clammy skin, c/o tightness in the chest with pain radiating to the left arm, BP 154/98, P. 100, R. 30. O_2 is at 2 L/nasal cannula, O_2 sat 88%.

Instructions: Based on the **10:00 AM**, identify and write the **priority problem** in the box below. Then, starting with the small box labeled **#1 prioritize** the **nursing interventions** for this situation and **identify** your follow-up action plan for Mrs. Tracey.

NURSING INTERVENTIONS | **DECISION-MAKING DIAGRAM**

A. Increase O_2 to 3 L

B. Raise to semi-Fowler's position

C. Administer nitroglycerin tab i q5min x3

D. Monitor vital signs q5min

E. Obtain a 12-lead EKG

F. Notify M.D.

New Action Plan

#1 #2 #3 #4 #5 #6

Priority Problem

NOTES

THE PATIENT WITH CHF

You are assigned to Mr. M. Tidwell who was transferred to your unit earlier today. In report you learn that he has CHF, 3+ pitting edema of the lower extremities, increasing SOB, has been demonstrating cheyne-stokes respirations, periods of confusion and c/o blurred vision.
VS are 97.6 - 62 - 22, BP 180/102. He has received his 0900 meds. Current orders include:

VS q4hrs I & O (✔) Up in chair qid O_2 @ 3 L/NP Serum K^+, PT, PTT, ABG (✔) Chest x-ray (✔) ECG (✔) Name: Tidwell, M. Age: 72	IV D5W @ 50 cc/hr IV site: LFA #20 g LBM: 2 days ago Foley (✔) Code Status: Full code Dx: CHF	Diet: Soft (NAS) Routine medications: Digoxin 0.25 mg IV q AM 09 Furosemide 40 mg po bid 09 -1700 Docusate sodium tab i po q AM 09 Minipress 10 mg po bid 09 -1700

Instructions: Prioritize the five **nursing interventions** as you would do them to take care of Mr. Tidwell. Write a number in the box to identify the order of your interventions (**#1** = first intervention, **#2** = second intervention, etc.) and state a **rationale** for each intervention.

INTERVENTIONS	PRIORITY #	RATIONALE
◇ Assess respiratory rate	1	
◇ Obtain urinary output data	4	
◇ Assess rate/rhythm and quality of pulse	2	
◇ Assess c/o visual disturbances	3	
◇ Check current lab data	5	

KEY POINTS TO CONSIDER:

Mr. Tidwell wants to wash up, but he says that he does not have the energy like he used to and that he gets tired very easily. You assess the following:

1) Skin cool, dusky in color
2) Lower extremities with 2+ pitting edema
3) Lung sounds with crackles on inspiration; resp. 24—regular pattern
4) Alert and oriented at this time

✓✓✓ **Interactive Activity:** With a partner, **do the following: (1) select** the **one nursing diagnosis** that is of priority at this time, **(2) provide a rationale** for your selection, and **(3) list the nursing interventions** that assist to meet the needs of the patient:

All of the following Nursing Diagnoses may apply to Mr. Tidwell.

Anxiety, Risk for infection, Activity intolerance, Fluid volume excess, Impaired tissue integrity, Risk for altered tissue perfusion: cerebral, Altered nutrition: Less than body requirements, Risk for injury, Knowledge deficit, Impaired gas exchange, Fatigue.

Nursing Diagnosis	Rationale	Nursing Interventions
		1. 2. 3. 4.

✓✓✓ Mr. Tidwell's family stops to visit during lunch. **At 1:00 PM,** the nursing assistant tells you that Mr. Tidwell is in distress. You walk into the room and notice Mr. Tidwell holding his chest tightly. Shortly after you assess:

cyanosis, no pulse, no BP and no respirations.

Instructions: Based on the **1:00 PM** situation, identify and write the **priority problem** in the box below. Then, starting with the small box labeled **#1 prioritize** the **nursing interventions** for this situation and **identify** your follow-up action plan for Mr. Tidwell.

NURSING INTERVENTIONS

A. Call a code

B. Place in supine position

C. Begin CPR

D. Document findings

E. Notify physician

F. Support family

DECISION-MAKING DIAGRAM

New Action Plan

#1 #2 #3 #4 #5 #6

Priority Problem

NOTES

THE PATIENT WITH A CVA

Mr. Henry, 68 yrs. old, suffered a right-sided CVA. He was admitted to the Telemety Unit 2 days ago and he has been on heparin therapy. The lastest documentation in the nursing notes shows: Hand grips R > L, speech slurred, BP 166/102. The orders in the nursing care kardex include:

VS q4hrs I & O (✔) Neuro checks q4hrs Up in chair today O_2 @ 2 L/NP Hospital day: #3	IV: 500 cc D_5W with heparin 10,000 u to infuse at 1000 U/hr Foley (✔) Foley care bid ROM to Left side Serum K^+, Na^+ & CBC today PTT daily	Diet: Full liquid Swallowing precautions Routine med: Docusate sodium 5 cc po qd Nimodipine 20 mg po tid

You begin your shift and during report you learn that Mr. Henry had a restful night and there were no changes in his condition. You prepare to assist Mr. Henry with his breakfast.

Instructions: Prioritize the five **nursing interventions** as you would do them to take care of Mr. Henry. Write a number in the box to identify the order of your interventions (**#1** = first intervention, **#2** = second intervention, etc.) and state a **rationale** for each intervention.

INTERVENTIONS	PRIORITY #	RATIONALE
◇ Position in high Fowler's	☐	______
◇ Place food on right side for patient to see	☐	______
◇ Place food into unaffected side of mouth	☐	______
◇ Check inside of mouth for food caught between gums and teeth (pocketing)	☐	______
◇ Use thick liquids	☐	______

KEY POINTS TO CONSIDER: ______

______

______

As morning care is given to Mr. Henry, you assess that he has the following:

1) Does not turn head if spoken to from left side
2) Left hand/arm elevated on a pillow
3) Passive ROM to left extremities
4) Antiembolism stockings on
5) Lack of awareness of left side

✓✓✓ **Interactive Activity:** With a partner, **do the following: (1) select** the **one nursing diagnosis** that is of priority at this time, **(2) provide a rationale** for your selection, and **(3) list the nursing interventions** that assist to meet the needs of the patient.

All of the following Nursing Diagnoses may apply to Mr. Henry.

Risk for injury: Fall, Knowledge deficit, Fear, Anxiety, Risk for infection, Impaired tissue integrity, Alteration in sensory/perceptual, Constipation, Impaired swallowing, Impaired verbal communication, Self-care deficit: bathing/hygiene, Altered urinary elimination pattern, Body image disturbance, Impaired physical mobility, Altered tissue perfusion, Risk for unilateral neglect, Risk for aspiration, Disuse Syndrome.

Nursing Diagnosis	Rationale	Nursing Interventions
		1. 2. 3.

✓✓✓ **Mr. Henry's lab** data is called to the unit. The results are:

PTT 200 secs. (control 38 secs.), K^+ 3.5 mEq, Na^+ 145 mEq, Hgb 11.4 g/dL, Hct 34%, Platelets 110,000/mm^3

Instructions: Based on **Mr. Henry's lab** data, identify and write the **priority problem** in the box below. Then, starting with the small box labeled **#1 prioritize** the **nursing interventions** for this situation and **identify** your follow-up action plan for Mr. Henry.

NURSING INTERVENTIONS

A. Notify physician

B. Prepare to administer protamine sulfate (if ordered)

C. Assess for petechiae

D. Monitor urine color

E. Monitor neuro status

F. Take the VS

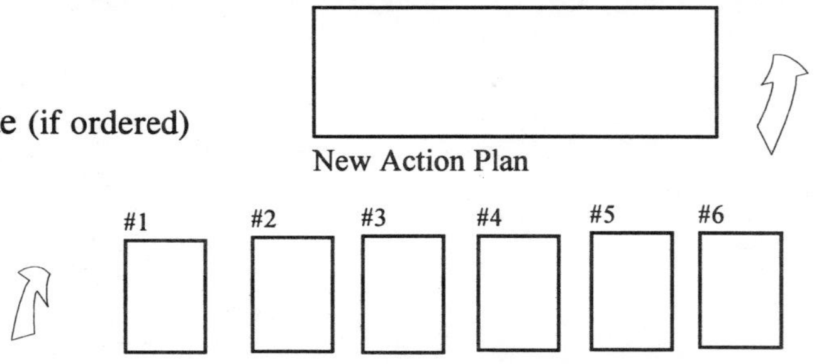

DECISION-MAKING DIAGRAM

New Action Plan

#1 #2 #3 #4 #5 #6

Priority Problem

NOTES

THE PATIENT WITH COPD

You are assigned to Mr. Troy, a 61-yr.-old male who has COPD. In the morning report you learn that he has been agitated during the night and is dyspneic this morning. The 0600 vital signs are 98.8 -102-32 BP 146/98. His 0700 pulse oximeter reading was 89% (room air) and he has an Aminophylline drip infusing at 6 mg/hr per controller and O_2 at 2 L/NC. He receives albuterol inhaler 2 puffs q4hrs and Atrovent inhaler 2 puffs q4hrs. He had a serum theophylline level drawn in the evening. You get out of report at 0730.

Instructions: Prioritize the five **nursing interventions** as you would do them to initially take care of Mr. Troy. Write a number in the box to identify the order of your interventions (**#1**=first intervention, **#2** = second intervention, etc.) and state a **rationale** for each intervention.

INTERVENTIONS	PRIORITY #	RATIONALE
◇ Auscultate lung sounds	3	
◇ Assess pulse oximeter, O_2 and NC	2	
◇ Retake the vital signs	4	
◇ Check theophylline level	5	
◇ Place in high Fowler's position	1	comfort

KEY POINTS TO CONSIDER: Baseline O_2 Sat & ↑ O_2 Pt. stop breathing, hypoxic drive, Pt. first ā lab work.

As you provide morning care to Mr. Troy you note the following signs and symptoms:

1) Nonproductive cough; long expiratory phase during respiration
2) Increased SOB c̄ mild exertion
3) Crackles audible throughout the bilateral lung fields
4) Anxious and restless
5) Theophylline level 14 μg/mL

✓✓✓ **Interactive Activity:** With a partner, **do the following: (1) select** the **one nursing diagnosis** that is of priority at this time, **(2) provide a rationale** for your selection, and **(3) list the nursing interventions** that assist to meet the needs of the patient:

All of the following Nursing Diagnoses may apply to Mr. Troy.

Ineffective breathing pattern, Ineffective airway clearance, Risk for injury, Infection Anxiety, Impaired gas exchange, Activity intolerance, Risk for impaired skin integrity, Altered nutrition: Less than body requirements, Sexual dysfunction.

Nursing Diagnosis	Rationale	Nursing Interventions
	COPD	1. 2. 3.

✓✓✓ At **12:00 PM** the patient care assistant reports that Mr. Troy is very warm and that his VS are 102-98-32 BP 140/84. He is expectorating thick, yellow-colored sputum.

Instructions: Based on the **12:00 PM** situation, identify and write the **priority problem** in the box below. Then, starting with the small box labeled **#1 prioritize** the **nursing interventions** for this situation and **identify** your follow-up action plan for Mr. Troy.

NURSING INTERVENTIONS

A. Auscultate lung sounds

B. Administer antipyretic if ordered

C. Provide cooling measures

D. Check O_2 saturation level

E. Retake vital signs in 2 hrs

F. Inform RN/physician

DECISION-MAKING DIAGRAM

New Action Plan: ↑ fluids, fever comfort measures

#1	#2	#3	#4	#5	#6
D	A	C	B	F	E

Priority Problem

NOTES

THE PATIENT WITH A CHEST TUBE

George, 23 yrs. old, has been in the hospital for two days after being stabbed in the chest. He has posterior chest tubes connected to a Pleu-evac system. You are assigned to his care and the nursing care kardex contains the following:

VS q4hrs I & O (✔) Amb with assist prn O_2 @ 2-3 L/NP/Pulse ox q4h Chest tube to low con't suction	IV: D5/0.45 NS q12 hrs IVPB cefazolin 1 g IV q6hrs Chest x-ray today ABG today	Diet: Soft Routine med: Colace 100 mg po qd

7:00 AM report indicates that he had a restful night. Chest tube drainage was 15 cc. Midnight VS are 99 - 90 - 22, BP 128/74. Pulse oximetry at 4:00 AM was 95%.

Instructions: Prioritize the five **nursing interventions** as you would do them to take care of George. Write a number in the box to identify the order of your interventions (**#1** = first intervention, **#2** = second intervention, etc.) and state a **rationale** for each intervention.

INTERVENTIONS	PRIORITY #	RATIONALE
◇ Check the pulse oximetry	☐	
◇ Assess for fluctuation in the water seal chamber & bubbling in the suction control chamber	☐	
◇ Check for the previous shift's fluid level marking on the tape	☐	
◇ Assess chest tube patency and drainage	☐	
◇ Ask George to cough and deep breathe	☐	

KEY POINTS TO CONSIDER:

After breakfast, George is transported to the x-ray department via wheelchair. Upon his return to his room you assess the following:

1) VS 99.8-92-26 BP 140/90
2) c/o dyspnea, crackles auscultated, anxious
3) O_2 off, O_2 saturation level 88%

✓✓✓ **Interactive Activity:** With a partner, **do the following: (1) select** the **one nursing diagnosis** that is of priority at this time, **(2) provide a rationale** for your selection, and **(3) list the nursing interventions** that assist to meet the needs of the patient:

All of the following Nursing Diagnoses may apply to George.

Ineffective airway clearance, Ineffective breathing pattern, Impaired gas exchange, Risk for injury, Knowledge deficit, Fear, Anxiety, Risk for infection, Impaired tissue integrity.

Nursing Diagnosis	Rationale	Nursing Interventions
		1. 2. 3. 4. 5.

✓✓✓ **One hour later,** George becomes increasingly restless and as you take his vital signs he pulls out the chest tube.

Instructions: Based on the **one hour later** situation, identify and write the **priority problem** in the box below. Then, starting with the small box labeled **#1 prioritize** the **nursing interventions** for this situation and **identify** your follow-up action plan for George.

NURSING INTERVENTIONS **DECISION-MAKING DIAGRAM**

A. Instruct George to take a deep breath and hold

B. Cover chest tube site with petroleum jelly and 4x4

C. Apply gloves

D. Increase O_2 to 3 L

E. Notify RN/physician

F. Pinch chest tube site together

New Action Plan

#1 #2 #3 #4 #5 #6

Priority Problem

NOTES____________________

THE PATIENT WITH UROSEPSIS

Mr. Tyler, 79 yrs. old, was admitted today to the hospital with the Dx. of Urosepsis. He has an IV of D5/0.45% NS infusing at 100 cc/hr. Rocephin 1 gm IVPB qd is ordered. He is on I & O q8hr, soft diet, BRP with assistance and Tylenol tabs $\overline{ii}$ p.o. q4h for temp >38. The day shift nurse indicated his VS were 38-78-22, BP 146/88 at 2:00 PM. The nurse also said that he was more restless this afternoon and had been trying to get out of bed and seemed somewhat disoriented. He did not receive Tylenol but an order for a vest restraint was obtained and has been applied. You have been assigned as his nurse for the evening shift.

Instructions: Prioritize the following **nursing interventions** as you, the nurse, would do them to initially take care of Mr. Tyler. Write a number in the box to identify the order of your interventions (**#1** = first intervention, **#2** = second intervention, etc.) and state a **rationale** for each intervention.

INTERVENTIONS	PRIORITY #	RATIONALE
◇ Administer Tylenol tabs $\overline{ii}$ p.o. if necessary		
◇ Take the vital signs		
◇ Gather urinary output data		
◇ Check the vest restraint		
◇ Perform a body systems physical assessment		

KEY POINTS TO CONSIDER:

You perform a follow-up assessment at 7:00 PM and note the following:

1) VS - 38.5 - 88 - 22, BP 120/76
2) Fine crackles audible on auscultation in the bilateral lower lung fields
3) He is sleepy.
4) He was incontinent of a scant amount of urine.

✓✓✓ **Interactive Activity:** With a partner, **do the following: (1) select** the **one nursing diagnosis** that is of priority at this time, **(2) provide a rationale** for your selection, and **(3) list the nursing interventions** that assist to meet the needs of the patient:

All of the following Nursing Diagnoses may apply to Mr. Tyler.

Risk for impaired skin integrity, Altered urinary elimination, Risk for injury, Altered thought processes, Hyperthermia, Fluid volume deficit, Altered nutrition: Less than body requirements, Ineffective breathing pattern, Fatigue.

Nursing Diagnosis	Rationale	Nursing Interventions
		1. 2. 3. 4. 5.

✓✓✓As you take his **8:00 PM** VS you note the following signs and symptoms on Mr. Tyler:

Lethargic, skin very warm and flushed, VS - 39.1 - 130 - 28, BP 90/54

Instructions: Based on the **8:00 PM** situation above, identify and write the **priority problem** in the box below. Then, starting with the small box labeled **#1 prioritize** the **nursing interventions** for this situation and **identify** your follow-up action plan for Mr. Tyler.

NURSING INTERVENTIONS

A. Check oxygen saturation level

B. Place in modified Trendelenburg position

C. Prepare to insert indwelling urinary catheter

D. Take vital signs

E. Document findings

F. Notify RN/physician

DECISION-MAKING DIAGRAM

New Action Plan

#1 #2 #3 #4 #5 #6

Priority Problem

NOTES

THE PATIENT WITH A TURP

Mr. Jacobs, 68 yrs. old, had a TURP this morning after having been diagnosed with benign prostatic hypertrophy. The following postop orders have been noted:

VS q4hr I & O qs Antiembolic hose x24 hrs Sequential TEDS x24 hrs Up in chair this pm	IV: RL @ 100 cc/hr IV site: RFA # 20 g 3-way urinary catheter to gravity c̄ continuous irrigation of NS to keep UA free of clots	Diet: Clear liquids this PM PRN Medication: B&O supp. q4hr prn bladder spasms

As you enter his room you notice that his urinary drainage bag is almost full and the Normal Saline irrigation bag is empty.

Instructions: Prioritize the five **nursing interventions** as you would do them to take care of Mr. Jacobs Write a number in the box to identify the order of your interventions (**#1** = first intervention, **#2** = second intervention, etc.) and state a **rationale** for each intervention.

INTERVENTIONS	PRIORITY #	RATIONALE
◊ Take the vital signs	☐	______
◊ Assess continuous urinary irrigation system	☐	______
◊ Empty urinary drainage bag	☐	______
◊ Perform a body systems physical assessment	☐	______
◊ Hang up new Normal saline irrigation bag	☐	______

KEY POINTS TO CONSIDER:______

______

______

The first postop day you assess the following on Mr. Jacobs:

1) VS: 99.6 - 88 - 20, 150/88
2) Urine pinkish, no clots
3) Grimaces and says "I didn't think it would be this tough."
4) Urinary catheter taped to thigh

✓✓✓ **Interactive Activity:** With a partner, **do the following: (1) select** the **one nursing diagnosis** that is of priority at this time, **(2) provide a rationale** for your selection, and **(3) list the nursing interventions** that assist to meet the needs of the patient:

All of the following Nursing Diagnoses may apply to Mr. Jacobs.

Risk for infection, Impaired tissue integrity, Risk for fluid volume excess, Knowledge deficit, Anxiety, Risk for injury: bleeding, Altered urinary elimination, Pain, Risk for altered sexuality pattern, Self-esteem disturbance, Altered tissue perfusion: peripheral.

Nursing Diagnosis	Rationale	Nursing Interventions
		1. 2. 3.

✓✓✓ The normal saline irrigation is discontinued at 12:00 PM the first postop day. Towards the end of the shift (**3:00 PM**), you **assess** the following on Mr. Jacobs:

c/o pain, no output since 12:00 PM, abdominal distention, and Mr. Jacobs is somewhat restless.

Instructions: Based on the **3:00 PM assessment** above, identify and write the **priority problem** in the box below. Then, starting with the small box labeled **#1 prioritize** the **nursing interventions** for this situation and **identify** your follow-up action plan for Mr. Jacobs.

NURSING INTERVENTIONS **DECISION-MAKING DIAGRAM**

A. Take the vital signs

B. Inform the RN/M.D.

C. Prepare to do a urinary irrigation

D. Give an antispasmotic

E. Place in low to semi-Fowler's position

F. Encourage fluids

New Action Plan

#1 #2 #3 #4 #5 #6

Priority Problem

NOTES____________________

THE PATIENT RECEIVING A BLOOD TRANSFUSION

Mr. Tanner, 34 yrs. old, was admitted for a motor vehicle accident: pedestrian vs car. He sustained multiple injuries throughout his body. He received two units of whole blood this morning. He has NS 0.9% infusing at TKO rate through a Y-shaped blood administration set and he has a 19 g cannula in the RFA. The M.D. orders to infuse each unit over 3-4 hours. As you get out of the report the lab notifies you that the first unit of blood is ready.

Instructions: Prioritize the five **nursing interventions** as you would do them to take care of Mr. Tanner. Write a number in the box to identify the order of your interventions (**#1** = first intervention, **#2** = second intervention, etc.) and state a **rationale** for each intervention.

INTERVENTIONS	PRIORITY #	RATIONALE
◇ Take an initial set of vital signs	☐	______
◇ Pick up the blood from the lab	☐	______
◇ Assess the IV site	☐	______
◇ Start the transfusion	☐	______
◇ Verify M.D. order, patient ID, & blood compatibility	☐	______

KEY POINTS TO CONSIDER:______

______

______

______

You assess the following during the start of the transfusion on Mr. Tanner:

1) VS: 97.6 - 80 - 18, BP 136/78 (pre-transfusion)
2) VS: 98.2 - 90 - 22, BP 130/70 (15 minutes after the start of the transfusion)
3) No complaints of itching
4) Transfusion rate increased to 100 cc/hr

✓✓✓ **Interactive Activity:** With a partner, **do the following: (1) select** the **one nursing diagnosis** that is of priority at this time, **(2) provide a rationale** for your selection, and **(3) list the nursing interventions** that assist to meet the needs of the patient:

All of the following Nursing Diagnoses may apply to Mr. Tanner.

Risk for infection, Anemia, Fatigue, Risk for fluid volume excess, Fluid volume deficit, Knowledge deficit, Anxiety, Risk for injury: blood administration, Pain.

Nursing Diagnosis	Rationale	Nursing Interventions
		1. 2. 3.

✓✓✓ After 20 minutes Mr. Tanner's **assessment** includes:

Skin flushed, P. 120, R. 32, BP 100/60, c/o chest pain and chills

Instructions: Based on the **assessment** above, identify and write the **priority problem** in the box below. Then, starting with the small box labeled **#1 prioritize** the **nursing interventions** for this situation and **identify** your follow-up action plan for Mr. Tanner.

NURSING INTERVENTIONS

A. Stop the transfusion

B. Inform RN/M.D.

C. Save next voided specimen

D. Start 0.9% NS at TKO rate

E. Take the vital signs

F. Save the transfusion unit

DECISION-MAKING DIAGRAM

New Action Plan

#1 #2 #3 #4 #5 #6

Priority Problem

NOTES

THE PATIENT WITH NEUTROPENIA

Mrs. K. Harvey, 50 yrs. old, was admitted two days ago with neutropenia. Her current WBC is 750/mm^3. During morning report you note the following from the nursing care kardex:

VS: q4hr I & O Neutropenic precautions (✔) Bone marrow biopsy—today CBC with diff—today Chest x-ray done	Diet: ↑ protein, ↑ calorie (no raw vegetables/fresh fruit) IV: D5W @ 125 cc/hr IV site: RFA (inserted 2 days ago)	Routine Medication: Colace 100 mg po qd PRN Medication: Tylenol 325 tabs ii q4h po prn temp >100.4

Instructions: Prioritize the five **nursing interventions** as you would do them to take care of Mrs. Harvey. Write a number in the box to identify the order of your interventions (**#1** = first intervention, **#2** = second intervention, etc.) and state a **rationale** for each intervention.

INTERVENTIONS	PRIORITY #	RATIONALE
◇ Wash hands	☐	___
◇ Assess the IV site	☐	___
◇ Provide fresh water at bedside	☐	___
◇ Assess oral mucosa	☐	___
◇ Take the vital signs	☐	___

KEY POINTS TO CONSIDER: ___

Mrs. Harvey is diagnosed with acute leukemia. Your follow-up assessment includes:

1) Hgb 9.8 g/dL, Hct 29%
2) WBC 900/mm^3
3) Using ordered antifungal medication as ordered
4) Platelet count 100,000/mm^3

✓✓✓ **Interactive Activity:** With a partner, **do the following: (1) select** the **one nursing diagnosis** that is of priority at this time, **(2) provide a rationale** for your selection, and **(3) list the nursing interventions** that assist to meet the needs of the patient:

All of the following Nursing Diagnoses may apply to Mrs. Harvey.

Risk for infection, Anemia, Fatigue, Altered nutrition: Less than body requirements, Knowledge deficit, Anxiety, Risk for injury: bleeding, Altered oral mucous membrane, Activity intolerance, Risk for impaired skin integrity, Social isolation, Risk for altered tissue perfusion.

Nursing Diagnosis	Rationale	Nursing Interventions
		1. 2. 3. 4.

✓✓✓ The following day, Mrs. Harvey's **assessment findings** are significant for:

Platelet count 30,000—Bleeding time prolonged, oral petechiae, hemoptysis, tachypnea, dyspnea, and a current nosebleed.

Instructions: Based on the **assessment** above, identify and write the **priority problem** in the box below. Then, starting with the small box labeled **#1 prioritize** the **nursing interventions** for this situation and **identify** your follow-up action plan for Mrs. Harvey.

NURSING INTERVENTIONS

A. Take the vital signs

B. Assess other sites for S & S of bleeding

C. Assess neuro status

D. Place in high Fowler's position

E. Apply direct pressure to nose

F. Inform RN/M.D.

Priority Problem

DECISION-MAKING DIAGRAM

New Action Plan

#1 #2 #3 #4 #5 #6

NOTES

THE PATIENT WITH A HIP FRACTURE

Mrs. Topps, 72 yrs. old, fell at home and was admitted to the hospital with a fracture of the right hip. She was alert and oriented upon admission. After the initial work up she was taken to surgery for an open reduction with internal fixation (ORIF) of her right hip. On her first postop day, her right hip dressing has a small amount of dried dark red drainage. She has an IV of D5/0.45% NS at 75 cc/hr, O_2 at 2 L/NP, clear liquid diet and circulation, movement, sensation, and temperature (CMST) neurovascular checks q4hr to the right leg for the first 24 hrs. The following medications are ordered: Meperidine 50 mg IM q3-4 hrs prn pain, $FeSo_4$ 325 mg p.o. tid with meals (start when on Regular diet), Colace 100 mg p.o. qd. She is very restless and confused this morning.

Instructions: Prioritize the five interventions according to Mrs. Topps current needs. Write a number in the box to identify the order of your interventions (**#1** = first intervention, **#2** = second intervention, etc.) and state a **rationale** for each intervention.

INTERVENTIONS	PRIORITY #	RATIONALE
◊ Assess surgical dressing		
◊ Take the vital signs	3	
◊ Assess pain level	2	
◊ Check O_2 saturation level	1	
◊ Check neurovascular status of right leg (CMST)		

KEY POINTS TO CONSIDER:

During the follow-up assessment for the **first postop day** you note the following:

1) Pedal pulse present, weak in the right foot; stronger on left foot
2) Hgb 10.5 g and Hct 32%
3) Bowel sounds hypoactive in all quadrants
4) Crackles in the lower bases of the lung

✓✓✓ **Interactive Activity:** With a partner, **do the following: (1) select** the **one nursing diagnosis** that is of priority at this time, **(2) provide a rationale** for your selection, and **(3) list three nursing interventions** that assist to meet the needs of the patient:

All of the following Nursing Diagnoses may apply to this Mrs. Topps.

Acute pain; Risk for infection; Risk for altered skin integrity; Altered patterns of elimination, Impaired gas exchange, Fatigue, Impaired physical mobility, Altered tissue perfusion: peripheral

Nursing Diagnosis	Rationale	Nursing Interventions
		1. 2. 3.

✓✓✓ On the second postop day Mrs. Topps is still very confused and is trying to get OOB. She has bilateral scattered crackles in the lungs, SOB on exertion, R. 32 and has a nonproductive cough.

Instructions: Based on the situation above, identify and write the **priority problem** in the box below. Then, starting with the small box labeled **#1 prioritize** the **nursing interventions** for this situation and **identify** your plan for follow-up care for Mrs. Topps.

NURSING INTERVENTIONS

A. Take vital signs

B. Check O_2 saturation

C. Stay with patient

D. Enc. incentive spirometer hourly

E. Call physician

F. Enc. fluids

DECISION-MAKING DIAGRAM

New Action Plan

#1 #2 #3 #4 #5 #6

Priority Problem

NOTES____________________

THE PATIENT WITH A FRACTURED TIBIA

Mr. F. Williams, 26 yrs. old, was admitted with a left fractured tibia. He was taken to surgery and is now being transferred to the Orthopedic Unit. He has a long leg cast on the left leg. His postop orders are transcribed to the nursing care kardex:

VS q4hrs I & O (✔) Neurovascular cks (circ. movement, sensation, temp) q4hr Elevate left leg on (1) pillow	1L D5W q10 hrs - dc when taking fluids well Teach crutch walking in AM	Diet: Clear liquids → Reg. PRN med: Meperidine 100 mg IM q4h prn pain

You are assigned to Mr. Williams as he is taken into his room. You note that he is alert, left leg cast is damp and clean, IV is infusing into right hand.

Instructions: Prioritize the five **nursing interventions** as you would do them to take care of Mr. Williams. Write a number in the box to identify the order of your interventions (**#1** = first intervention, **#2** = second intervention, etc.) and state a **rationale** for each intervention.

INTERVENTIONS	PRIORITY #	RATIONALE
◇ Take the vital signs	☐	______
◇ Neurovascular assessment of both extremities	☐	______
◇ Assess cast for dryness, signs of drainage and sharp edges	☐	______
◇ Use palms of hands to elevate cast on a pillow	☐	______
◇ Apply sterile dressing to left foot	☐	______

KEY POINTS TO CONSIDER: ______

On the morning of the first postop day, you note that Mr. Williams is:

1) Requesting pain med q4hrs
2) Left pedal pulses present, edema 2+
3) Capillary refill >2 sec, moves left toes
4) Taking fluids and voiding qs
5) M.D. orders CPK, LDH, and SGOT

✓✓✓ **Interactive Activity:** With a partner, **do the following: (1) select** the **one nursing diagnosis** that is of priority at this time, **(2) provide a rationale** for your selection, and **(3) list the nursing interventions** that assist to meet the needs of the patient.

All of the following Nursing Diagnoses may apply to Mr. Williams.

Risk for injury, Knowledge deficit, Risk for infection, Risk for impaired skin integrity, Risk for impaired physical mobility, Fear, Altered tissue perfusion: peripheral, Pain, Activity intolerance, Impaired tissue integrity, Anxiety, Risk for peripheral neurovascular dysfunction.

Nursing Diagnosis	Rationale	Nursing Interventions
		1. 2. 3.

✓✓✓ **Mr. Williams refuses lunch** and you assess:

c/o increased pain, esp. with elevation of leg, numbness and tingling, left pedal pulse weak, cool

Instructions: Based on **Mr. Williams refuses lunch** information, identify and write the **priority problem** in the box below. Then, starting with the small box labeled **#1 prioritize** the **nursing interventions** for this situation and **identify** your follow-up action plan for Mr. Williams.

NURSING INTERVENTIONS

A. Inform RN/M.D. stat

B. Prepare to have cast bivalved

C. Ensure left extremity is at heart level

D. Monitor left pedal pulse

E. Take the vital signs

F. Stay with patient

DECISION-MAKING DIAGRAM

New Action Plan

#1 #2 #3 #4 #5 #6

Priority Problem

NOTES

THE PATIENT WITH CATARACT SURGERY

Mrs. Tami Fields, 72 yrs. old, has senile cataracts and has been instilling mydriatic eye gtts. Her vision has progressively worsened and she is scheduled today for a right cataract extraction in the outpatient clinic. The M.D. orders the following preop preparation: NPO, instill myriatic and cyclopegic eye gtts 1 hour prior to surgery, Valium 5 mg po 1 hour prior to surgery. Mrs. Fields arrives at the outpatient clinic at 0800 and she is scheduled for surgery at 1000.

Instructions: Prioritize the five **nursing interventions** as you would do them to take care of Mrs. Fields. Write a number in the box to identify the order of your interventions (**#1** = first intervention, **#2** = second intervention, etc.) and state a **rationale** for each intervention.

INTERVENTIONS	PRIORITY #	RATIONALE
◇ Provide information regarding preop preparation	☐	____________________
◇ Begin to instill ordered eye gtts	☐	____________________
◇ Have patient void	☐	____________________
◇ Take the vital signs	☐	____________________
◇ Ensure the surgical consent is signed	☐	____________________

KEY POINTS TO CONSIDER: ____________________

Mrs. Fields had an intraocular lens implant and is taken to the recovery room. She has an eye patch on her right eye and you assess the following:

1) No c/o pain, P. 88, BP 130/82
2) Eye patch clean and dry
3) Readily responds to verbal stimuli

✓✓✓ **Interactive Activity:** With a partner, **do the following: (1) select** the **one nursing diagnosis** that is of priority at this time, **(2) provide a rationale** for your selection, and **(3) list the nursing interventions** that assist to meet the needs of the patient:

All of the following Nursing Diagnoses may apply to Mrs. Fields.

Risk for injury, Knowledge deficit, Sensory-perceptual alterations; visual, Fear, Anxiety, Risk for self-care deficit, Risk for infection, Altered health maintenance, Impaired home maintenance management.

Nursing Diagnosis	Rationale	Nursing Interventions
		1. 2. 3.

✓✓✓ One hour **postop** you assess Mrs. Fields and note the following:

c/o right brow pain, anxious, P. 110, BP 128/80 coughing and c/o nausea

Instructions: Based on the **postop** assessment, identify and write the **priority problem** in the box below. Then, starting with the small box labeled **#1 prioritize** the **nursing interventions** for this situation and **identify** your follow-up action plan for Mrs. Fields.

NURSING INTERVENTIONS

A. Avoid rapid head movement

B. Administered antiemetic if ordered

C. Document findings/nursing care

D. Notify M.D.

E. Recheck pulse and BP

F. Stay with Mrs. Fields

DECISION-MAKING DIAGRAM

New Action Plan

#1 #2 #3 #4 #5 #6

Priority Problem

NOTES

THE PATIENT WITH A SEIZURE DISORDER

Mr. Michaels, 20 yrs. old, fell at home and was brought to the emergency room after it was noticed that he had lost consciousness for a few seconds. In the emergency room he indicated that he did not remember falling. His family history is significant for seizure disorders. Diagnostic studies were ordered and included an EEG, MRI, serum fasting blood sugar, CBC, BUN, and UA drug screening. He was just transferred to the neurological unit from the emergency room. The current M.D. orders include: seizure precautions, bedrest, soft diet, saline lock, and vital signs and neuro checks q4hrs.

Instructions: Prioritize the following **nursing interventions** as you would do them to initially take care of Mr. Michaels. Write a number in the box to identify the order of your interventions (**#1** = first intervention, **#2** = second intervention, etc.) and state a **rationale** for each intervention.

INTERVENTIONS	PRIORITY #	RATIONALE
◇ Orient Mr. Michaels to his room	☐	
◇ Assess neurological status	☐	
◇ Implement seizure precautions	☐	
◇ Obtain admitting history	☐	
◇ Inform of pertinent M.D. orders	☐	

KEY POINTS TO CONSIDER:

Mr. Michaels is diagnosed with a seizure disorder and is started on Depakote. In speaking with Mr. Michaels you gather the following:

1) Mr. Michaels says that he has had similar episodes but never told anyone
2) He remembers seeing "spots" before the episode
3) No one in his family talked much about the relative who had seizures

✓✓✓ **Interactive Activity:** With a partner, **do the following: (1) select** the **one nursing diagnosis** that is of priority at this time, **(2) provide a rationale** for your selection, and **(3) list the nursing interventions** that assist to meet the needs of the patient:

All of the following Nursing Diagnoses may apply to Mr. Michaels.

Ineffective individual coping, Ineffective airway clearance, Risk for injury, Knowledge deficit, Self-esteem disturbance, Social isolation, Fear, Anxiety, Altered thought processes, Risk for aspiration.

Nursing Diagnosis	Rationale	Nursing Interventions
		1. 2. 3.

✓✓✓ Several hours after admission, you hear a "cry" coming from Mr. Michaels' room. You assess the following as you walk into the room:

Tonic-clonic movements of the body, loss of consciousness, excessive salivation, some cyanosis, urinary incontinence, teeth clenched with cessation of tonic-clonic movements after 3 minutes.

Instructions: Based on the situation above, identify and write the **priority problem** in the box below. Then, starting with the small box labeled **#1 prioritize** the **nursing interventions** for this situation and **identify** your follow-up action plan for Mr. Michaels.

NURSING INTERVENTIONS

A. Maintain a quiet environment

B. Assess for injury

C. Check airway patency

D. Document findings

E. Turn to side

F. Reorient patient

DECISION-MAKING DIAGRAM

New Action Plan

#1 #2 #3 #4 #5 #6

Priority Problem

NOTES

THE PATIENT WITH A DNR ORDER

Mr. Bala, 83 yrs. old, has terminal esophageal cancer. The following pertinent information is found in the nursing care kardex:

Activity: Bedrest Vital signs: q4hrs O_2 sats: q4hr Lives with son Hospital Day: #4	PEG tube insertion: 3 days ago Formula full strength - 50 cc/hr Ck residual q4hrs, if > 100 cc hold feeding for 1 hour MS 2 mg IV q2hrs prn pain	IV: D5/0.45 NS q12hrs Urinary catheter inserted on admission I & O q8hrs Code Status: No code

The 7:00 AM report indicates that his current respirations are 10 and he last received MS at 6:00 AM. Residual at that time was 125 cc—tube feeding was stopped. IV has 200 cc left.

Instructions: Prioritize the five **nursing interventions** as you would do them to initially take care of Mr. Bala Write a number in the box to identify the order of your interventions (**#1**= first intervention, **#2** = second intervention, etc.) and state a **rationale** for each intervention.

INTERVENTIONS	PRIORITY #	RATIONALE
◇ Assess PEG tube residual	☐	______
◇ Take the vital signs	☐	______
◇ Assess IV site and IV fluid level	☐	______
◇ Perform a body system's assessment	☐	______
◇ Assess O_2 saturation level	☐	______

KEY POINTS TO CONSIDER: ______

At 11:00 AM Mr. Bala manifested the following signs and symptoms:

1) VS: pulse 76, resp. 14, BP 118/64
2) Responds appropriately, but is weak and lethargic
3) Urine is dark yellow; output 125 cc since 7:00 AM
4) SOB when turning; irregular breathing pattern

✓✓✓ **Interactive Activity:** With a partner, **do the following: (1) based on the current assessment, select** the **one nursing diagnosis** that is of priority at this time, **(2) provide a rationale** for your selection, and **(3) list three nursing interventions** that meet the needs of the patient:

All of the following Nursing Diagnoses may apply to Mr. Bala.

Risk for infection, Pain, Anxiety, Impaired gas exchange, Altered nutrition: Less than body requirements, Risk for fluid volume deficit, Risk for impaired skin integrity, Altered tissue perfusion, Activity Intolerance, Powerlessness, Social Isolation.

Nursing Diagnosis	Rationale	Nursing Interventions
		1. 2. 3.

✓✓✓ At **2:00 PM** Mr. Bala is unresponsive to verbal stimuli. You assessed:

VS: pulse 36, resp. 9, BP 80/50. Urine output unchanged since 11:00 AM. Lower extremeties cool with cyanosis.

Instructions: Based on the **2:00 PM** assessment, identify and write the **priority problem** in the box below. Then, starting with the small box labeled **#1 prioritize** the **nursing interventions** for this situation and **identify** your plan for follow-up care for Mr. Bala.

NURSING INTERVENTIONS

A. Monitor P., R., and BP

B. Check NCP for religious/cultural requests

C. Report findings to RN

D. Notify relatives

E. Provide comfort measures

F. Document findings

DECISION-MAKING DIAGRAM

New Action Plan

#1 #2 #3 #4 #5 #6

Priority Problem

NOTES

LEGAL CONSIDERATIONS

Mrs. Lyle is one day postop total abdominal hysterectomy. She is 42 yrs. old. Demerol 75 mg is ordered IM q3hrs prn pain. She is on a clear liquid diet and has not voided since the urinary catheter was removed at noon. She is ambulating with assistance to the bathroom. The abdominal dressing is stained with dried dark red drainage. Noon vital signs are 99 - 82 - 22 and BP 130/76. Fine crackles are audible in the lower bases of the lung fields. It is 4:00 PM and she is requesting pain medication. Her last pain shot was administered at 2:00 PM. Incentive spirometer is at bedside.

Instructions: Prioritize the following **nursing interventions** as you, the nurse, would do them to initially take care of Mrs. Lyle. Write a number in the box to identify the order of your interventions (**#1** = first intervention, **#2** = second intervention, etc.) and state a **rationale** for each intervention.

INTERVENTIONS	PRIORITY #	RATIONALE
◇ Inform Mrs. Lyle that the pain medication is not due for another hour	☐	______
◇ Cough and deep breath; demonstrate abdominal splinting. Use incentive spirometer q1h	☐	______
◇ Ambulate to the bathroom	☐	______
◇ Take the vital signs	☐	______
◇ Assess abdomen and surgical dressing	☐	______

KEY POINTS TO CONSIDER: ______

Mrs. Lyle voids 400 cc after ambulating to the bathroom and states that she feels much better. She relates the following to you:

1) Her mother had a hysterectomy, but died 10 days after from surgical complications.
2) She is glad that she does not have to worry about irregular periods anymore.
3) She fully trusts her doctor but wonders whether the right thing was done.
4) She lives alone.

✓✓✓ **Interactive Activity:** With a partner, **do the following: (1) based on the current assessment, select** the **one nursing diagnosis** that is of priority at this time, **(2) provide a rationale** for your selection, and **(3) list three nursing interventions** that meet the needs of the patient:

All of the following Nursing Diagnoses may apply to Mrs. Lyle.

Risk for infection, Pain, Anxiety, Ineffective breathing pattern, Altered nutrition: Less than body requirements, Body image disturbance, Risk for sexual dysfunction, Impaired skin integrity, Risk for activity intolerance, Knowledge deficit.

Nursing Diagnosis	Rationale	Nursing Interventions
		1. 2. 3.

✓✓✓ At 6:00 PM Mrs. Lyle states that she is having pain. In fact on a scale from 1-10, Mrs. Lyle's pain is an 8. She has not received any pain medication since 2:00 PM.

You take out an ampule labeled Demerol 100 mg/ml and administer 1 mL.
Mrs. Lyle asks whether the 75 mg of Demerol would help her since it did not help her before.

Instructions: Based on the situation above, identify and write the **priority problem** in the box below. Then, starting with the small box labeled **#1 prioritize** the **nursing interventions** for this situation and **identify** your follow-up action plan for Mrs. Lyle.

NURSING INTERVENTIONS **DECISION-MAKING DIAGRAM**

A. Tell pt. you administered 100 mg of Demerol

B. Document drug and amount given

C. Monitor P., R., and BP

D. Fill out an incident report

E. Notify your instructor

F. Notify physician

New Action Plan

#1 #2 #3 #4 #5 #6

Priority Problem

NOTES____________________

SECTION THREE

Applying the Critical Thinking Model

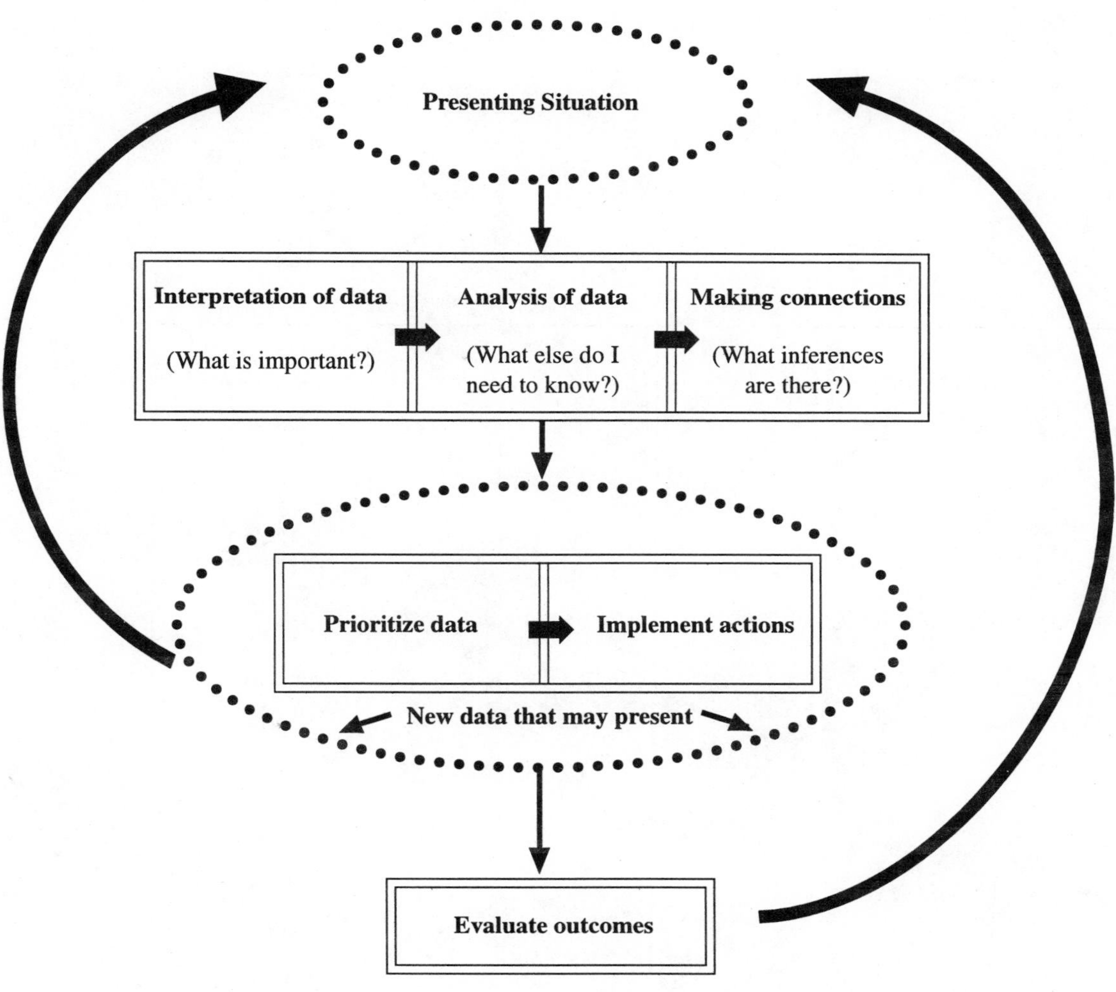

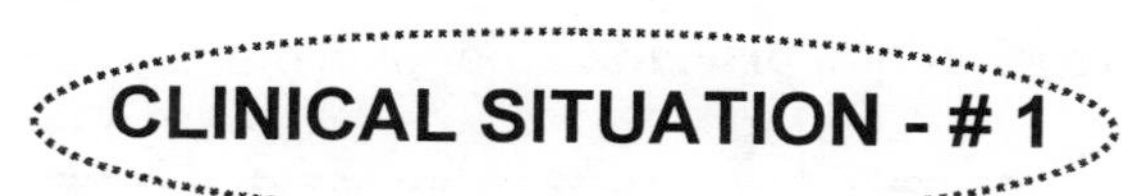

Intershift taped report at 0700:

"Mr. Andrews, 72 yrs. old, is 2 days postop small bowel resection. His N/G tube is connected to low wall suction and is draining dark brown fluid. Vital signs at 0600: 99.6 - 90 - 28 160/94. IV D_5/0.45% NS with 20 mEq KCl infusing at 125 cc into the right forearm. He is using the PCA machine. He slept most of the night and is now sitting in a chair. SOB was noted when he was transferred to the chair. There are 300 cc's left in the IV."

Mr. Andrews' current **flow charts** contain the following information:

Medication Record

Routine	**Time Due**
Lanoxin 0.25 mg IV qd	0900
Lasix 20 mg IVP qd	0900
Timolol 0.25% gtt ī OU bid	1000
Zantac 50 mg IVPB q6h	1000
Gentamicin 80 mg IVPB q8h	1400

PRN

Phenergan 25 mg IV/IM q4h pr N/V
PCA (morphine sulfate - 1 mg/hr)

Intake and Output Record

Night Shift @ 0600

Intake		**Output**	
P.O.	= 0	UA void	= 0
		Foley	= 200
IV	= 1000	N/G	= 600
IVPB	= 100		

Interactive Activity: With a partner, **use the case study and the flow charts** to:

1. Identify the pertinent patient information made known to you in the report	2. Identify the pertinent information you gathered from the flow charts	3. Review the data in columns 1 & 2 and identify information that needs follow-up

It is 0730 as you leave the report room, **prioritize** your plan of care for the morning:

Time	Plan of Nursing Care

1200 nursing assessment: Oriented x3, skin WNL, capillary refill < 3 sec., turgor good, mucous membranes moist, pinkish, T. 99, P. 88 slightly irregular, R. 24, BP 164/94. N/G draining brownish fluid 100 cc since 0800. Bowel sounds present x4, abd. soft. Foley catheter draining clear yellow urine.

Mr. Andrews has minimal complaints and is visited by the physician at 1200. The physician leaves the following orders:

Remove Foley now
Enc. incentive spirometer q1h x10
Discontinue N/G tube
DC Lasix
Lanoxin 0.25 mg po qd
Hgb & Hct today
Clear liquid diet

1. Identify the nursing interventions that require immediate follow-up	2. Identify the nursing actions that you can delegate/assign to unlicensed personnel

For each of the following **nursing interventions**, write an **expected patient outcome**:

1. Foley removed at 1300 ⇨
2. Incentive spirometer q1h x10 ⇨

CLINICAL SITUATION - # 2

Intershift taped report at 7:00 a.m.:

"Mr. Forsthworth, 43 yrs. old, was admitted 2 nights ago after experiencing GI bleed. He is NPO and has an N/G tube connected to continuous suction. The N/G has drained 100 cc of dark reddish drainage. Vital signs at 6:00 AM are 97.4 - 96 -18 130/86. A unit of whole blood is infusing and should be complete by 9:00 AM. His current Hgb is 8.6. He does have a history of ETOH abuse and has been more restless this morning."

Mr. Forsthworth's current **flow charts** contain the following information:

Patient Care Kardex

IV: D5/0.9% NS c̄ 10 cc MVI @ 100 cc/hr

IV site: #18 g LFA; saline lock RFA#20 g

Give two units of whole blood today ☑ ☐
H & H in the AM

Routine Medication:
Mylanta 30 cc q4h/NG (Clamp tube for 30 min p̄ administration)
Tagamet 300 mg IVPB q6h 10-4-10-4

Intake and Output Record

Night Shift @ 0600

Intake		**Output**	
P.O.	= 0	UA void	= 525
		N/G	= 100
IV	= 600		
0.9% NS	= 50		
Tranfusion	= 50		

Interactive Activity: With a partner, **use the case study and the flow charts** to:

1. Identify the pertinent patient information made known to you in the <u>report</u>	2. Identify the pertinent information you gathered from the <u>flow charts</u>	3. Review the data in columns 1 & 2 and identify information that needs follow-up

It is 7:30 AM as you leave the report room, **prioritize** your plan of care for the morning:

Time	Plan of Nursing Care

10:00 AM nursing assessment: Anxious, restless, pulled out N/G tube. Physician called. Wrist restraints applied. VS: P. 100, R. 24, BP 146/90. Vomited 20 cc bright red fluid. Bowel sounds present x4, abd. soft. Transfusion #2 infusing at 25 gtt/min.

The physician calls back and gives the following telephone orders:

Wrist and vest posey restraints prn
Oxygen at 2L/min/NP
Reinsert N/G tube
ABG, serum electrolytes Mg^{++}, BS, H & H
VS and neuro checks q2hrs
Librium 50 mg IM q3h prn restlessness
Phenergan 25 mg IM q4hr prn N/V

1. Identify the nursing interventions that require immediate follow-up	**2. Identify the nursing actions that you can delegate/assign to unlicensed personnel**

For each of the following **nursing interventions**, write **expected patient outcomes**:

1. Application of wrist and vest posey ⇨

2. Librium 50 mg IM ⇨

CLINICAL SITUATION - # 3

Intershift taped report at 1600:

"Mrs. Gilroy, 88 yrs. old, was admitted today with dehydration. She has a Stage IV pressure ulcer on her sacrum. A wet to dry dressing was applied. A pressure ulcer with eschar is on her left heel. She weighs 90 lb. and she refused her lunch. An IV was started at 1400. You have 750 cc credit. She is a sweet little lady, quiet and at times forgetful. Her admission lab results just came in, her Hgb is 9.6, Hct 27, WBC 11,000 and K^+ 4.5. I have not called the physician."

Mrs. Gilroy 's current **flow charts** contain the following information:

Patient Care Kardex

VS q4h — Diet: Pureed
HOH
Siderails ↑ at all times
W-D Drsg c̄ 0.9 NS 0600-1400-2200

IV: D5/0.9 NS at 75 cc/hr
IV site: R hand #24 g cannula

Medication: Colace 100 mg qd

NO CODE

Intake and Output Record
Day Shift - 8 hour

Intake	Output
P.O. = 50	UA = inc x2
IV = 250	

Interactive Activity: With a partner, **use the case study and the flow charts** to:

1. Identify the pertinent patient information made known to you in the report	2. Identify the pertinent information you gathered from the flow charts	3. Review the data in columns 1 & 2 and identify information that needs follow-up

It is 1630 as you leave the report room, **prioritize** your plan of care for the next four hours:

Time	Plan of Nursing Care

At 2000 the nursing assistant reports that Mrs. Gilroy is restless and trying to get out of bed. You document the following assessment: Speech incoherent, skin warm, flushed. VS: 101-92-24 108/60. Incontinent of dark-colored urine with strong odor. Physician called.

The following telephone orders are given:

Catheterize for post-residual urine
VS q2h, I & O
Tylenol 325 mg po q4h prn T. > 100.4
Vest posey restraint prn
Enc. fluid intake
Rocephin 1 g IVPB qd

1. Identify the nursing interventions that require immediate follow-up	2. Identify the nursing actions that you can delegate/assign to unlicensed personnel

For the following **nursing intervention**, write an **expected patient outcome:**

1. Monitor I & O q8hrs ⇨

CLINICAL SITUATION - # 4

Intershift taped report at 2300:

"Mr. Jackson was admitted with a fractured right tibia and is one day postop. He has a cast on. He has been quiet most of the evening. He has just started coughing and is experiencing some SOB. He says he has a history of asthma and he says that he gets this way every now and then. I did not detect any wheezing. Vital signs are 98.8 - 90 - 28 140/88. Circulation, movement, and sensation are WNL in the right leg."

Mr. Jackson's current **flow charts** contain the following information:

Nursing Care Rand

Diet: Regular

Up in chair
PT to teach crutch walking ☑

IV: Saline lock #20 g RFA

Circ. movement, sensation and temp. (CMST) ® leg q4h
Elevate leg on one pillow

PRN Medication:
Meperidine HCL 75 mg IM q3-4 hr prn pain

Medical History

Smokes ½ -1 pack of cigarettes/day

Respiratory infection 1 month ago
Uses cromolyn inhaler prn

CBC WNL } Day of admission
ESR ↑

G. Jackson 48-yr.-old male.

Interactive Activity: With a partner, **use the case study and the flow charts** to:

1. Identify the pertinent patient information made known to you in the report	2. Identify the pertinent information you gathered from the flow charts	3. Review the data in columns 1 & 2 and identify information that needs follow-up

It is 2330 as you leave the report room, **prioritize** your plan of care for the next 3 hours:

Time	Plan of Nursing Care

0200 nursing assessment: Mr. Jackson is beginning to cough more frequently, c/o chest tightness. Respiratory assessment indicates inspiratory and expiratory wheezes in bilateral lungs. You call the physician and obtain the following telephone orders.

IV D5/0.9 NS at 125 cc/hr
Oxygen at 2 L/NP
Ventolin inhaler 2 puffs q4h
Alupent nebulizer treatment q3hr
ABG, Sputum for eosinophils
Solu-Medrol 125 mg IVP q6h
Check oxygen saturation with pulse oximeter q2h
Call physician with ABG results

1. Identify the nursing interventions that require immediate follow-up	2. Identify the nursing actions that you can delegate/assign to unlicensed personnel

For each of the following **nursing interventions**, write an **expected patient outcome**:

1. Alupent treatment q3hrs ⇨
2. Solu-medrol 125 mg IVP ⇨

CLINICAL SITUATION - # 5

Intershift taped report at 3:00 PM:

"Mrs. Clark, 42 yrs. old, was admitted earlier today with acute pancreatitis. She had mid-epigastric pain with nausea and vomiting on admission. Her latest vitals signs are 38 - 108 - 26, 110/60. Bowel sounds are hypoactive. I medicated her at 2:00 PM. A central line was inserted, you have 800 cc left in the IV. The N/G is draining brownish fluid. She needs to have the urinary catheter inserted."

Mrs. Clark's current **flow charts** contain the following information:

Patient Care Kardex

VS: q4hrs Diet: NPO
O2 @ 3 L/NP
Pulse oximetry q4hrs

IV: D_5W @125 cc/hr
Right central line
N/G tube to low con't suction ☑
Urinary catheter inserted ☐

ABG in AM ☐
K^+, Na^+, Cl^-, CO_2, Mg^{2+}, Ca^{++} in AM ☐
Abd CT scan @ 6 PM today

Routine Medication:
Cimetidine 300 mg IVPB q6h 10-4-10-4

PRN Medication:
Meperidine 75 mg IM q3h prn pain

Admission Lab Data

Se Amylase 350 units/L
Se Lipase 260 units/L

Hgb 11.6 g/dL
Hct 32%
WBC 18,000/mm^3

LDH 300 units/L
AST 80 units/L

BS 200 mg/dL

Interactive Activity: With a partner, **use the case study and the flow charts** to:

1. Identify the pertinent patient information made known to you in the report	2. Identify the pertinent information you gathered from the flow charts	3. Review the data in columns 1 & 2 and identify information that needs follow-up

It is 4:00 PM, prioritize your plan of care for the next three hours:

Time	Plan of Nursing Care

At 8:30 PM the nursing assistant informs you that Mrs. Clark is complaining of pain and is restless. You note that she has not had a pain shot in the last three hours. You walk into the room to assess her and to give her a meperidine injection. She turns over quickly and pulls out the central line.

1. Identify the nursing interventions that you would implement immediately at the bedside.	**2. Identify the follow-up nursing actions. Document the incident in the nurse's notes.**

Nurse's Notes

For the following **nursing intervention**, write the **expected patient outcome**:

1. Call physician regarding abnormal lab values ⇨

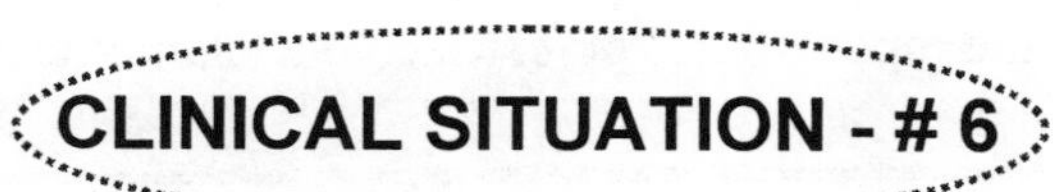

CLINICAL SITUATION - # 6

Intershift taped report at 8:00 a.m.:

"Timmy Wiley was been transferred from the ICU yesterday. He was in an MVA fourteen days ago. He had some head trauma and subsequent evacuation of a subdural hematoma. He is unconscious, unresponsive to painful stimuli and flaccid. Pupils sluggish. He has several abrasions on his face and several bruised areas on his shoulders and chest from the accident. Vital signs are 97.8 -94-24, BP 124/80. Mother at bedside, she questions everything you do."

Timmy's current **flow charts** contain the following information:

Nursing Care Rand

Suction prn Diet: NPO
VS & Neuro checks q4hrs
Seizure precautions Foley ☑
HOB ↑ 30° at all times I & O
LBM: ______ PEG tube clamped
IV: D5/0.9% NS @ 100 cc/ hr via ® central line
Fingerstick BS q6h 12-6-12-6

Routine Medication:

Decadron 4 mg IVP 10-4-10-4
Dulcolax supp. prn

Medical History

18-year-old high school student involved a MVA in which he was the driver. Passenger in the car died from the injuries.
Pt. unconscious on arrival to the ER.

Drug use: Family not aware of any use.
Blood alcohol level on admission 0.16%

Family wants to continue all possible treatment. Not willing to discuss code status at this time.

Interactive Activity: With a partner, **use the case study and the flow charts** to:

1. Identify the pertinent patient information made known to you in the report	2. Identify the pertinent information you gathered from the flow charts	3. Review the data in columns 1 & 2 and identify information that needs follow-up

It is 8:30 AM as you leave the report room, **prioritize** your plan of care for the next 3 hours:

Time	Plan of Nursing Care

2:00 PM nursing assessment: Pupil R • L ● Resp. 12 Cheyne-Stokes. Pulse 80, BP 150/80. Skin warm, jerky movements of the upper extremity noted.

The physician writes the following orders:

Oxygen at 2 L/NP
Check oxygen saturation q1h
Vital signs q1h
CT scan stat
ABGs stat

1. Identify the nursing interventions that require immediate follow-up	2. Identify the nursing actions that you can delegate/assign to unlicensed personnel

For each of the following **nursing interventions**, write **expected patient outcomes**:

1. Oxygen 2 L/NP ⇨
2. Seizure precautions ⇨

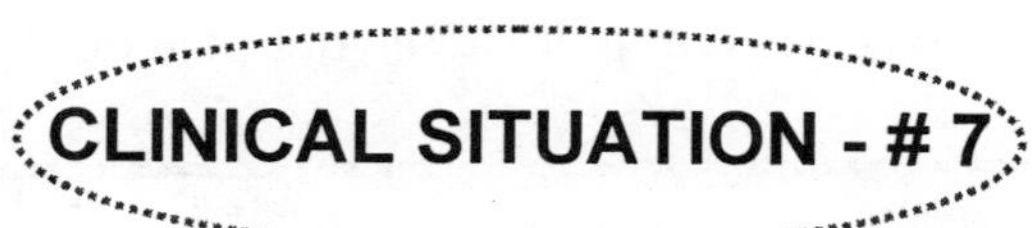

CLINICAL SITUATION - # 7

Intershift taped report at 8:00 AM:

"Mrs. Brown is 52 yrs. old with bone cancer. She has been requesting pain medication every two hours. I gave her MS 2 mg this morning at 6:30 AM. Her respirations have gone down to ten during the night. She does not want to be turned. A urinary catheter was inserted in the evening shift. She is a no code. A family member spent the night with her. Latest vital signs at 6:00 AM are 97-66-12, 128/60."

Mrs. Brown's current **flow charts** contain the following information:

Nursing Care Rand

Diet: DAT
VS q4hrs
Foley ☑
Comfort measures I & O
IV: Saline lock
LBM: inc. x1 sml

PRN Medication:
MS 2 mg IV q2hr prn
MS 4 mg IV q2hr prn if not relieved with MS 2 mg
No code

Nurse's Notes

Night shift
11:00 PM Awake, responds when spoken to c/o generalized pain, refuses to be turned. Medicated with MS 2 mg IV. *C. Todd RN*
11:30 Resp 10, moans when touched, taking sips of water. Mouth care given. *C. Todd RN*
12:00 AM Moaning. Daughter upset, crying states is afraid that mother is going to die. Referral to pastoral care given. *C. Todd RN*
1:00 MS 2 mg given IV, lethargic, arouse-able resp. 10, P. 60 BP 110/58. *C. Todd RN*
4:30 Pain med given with relief. *C. Todd RN*

Interactive Activity: With a partner, **use the case study and the flow charts** to:

1. Identify the pertinent patient information made known to you in the <u>report</u>	2. Identify the pertinent information you gathered from the <u>flow charts</u>	3. Review the data in columns 1 & 2 and identify information that needs follow-up

It is 8:30 AM as you leave the report room, **prioritize** your plan of care for the next 3 hours:

Time	**Plan of Nursing Care**

At 12:30 PM you return from lunch to learn that the nursing assistant was unable to obtain a pulse on Mrs. Brown. You assess the following: unresponsive, skin cool, legs pale with mottling. Pulse not palpable, no apical or BP audible. Family with patient. Physician contacted and pronounced patient deceased.

Family is making arrangements for a mortuary to pick up Mrs. Brown within the hour.

1. Identify the nursing interventions that require immediate follow-up	**2. Identify the nursing actions that you can delegate/assign to unlicensed personnel**

For each of the following **nursing interventions**, write an **expected outcome**:

1. Provide postmortem care ⇨ ______

2. Speak with family ⇨ ______

CLINICAL SITUATION - # 8

Intershift taped report at 7:00 AM:

"Mrs. Fritz, 79 yrs. old, was in a motor vehicle accident two days ago in which she fractured her arm. Her right arm is in a cast, circulation, movement, and sensation is fine. She is scheduled to go home this morning, she slept fine and was medicated for pain once during the night with relief."

"**At 7:30 AM**, as you are coming out of report, the night nurse tells you that Mrs. Fritz got up to go to the bathroom and fell coming back to bed. She has a slight nosebleed, was given an icepack and assisted back to bed. The physician was called and informed of her falling. He said he will be in later to see her before discharge. No new orders were given."

Mrs. Fritz's current **flow charts** contain the following information:

Nursing Care Rand

VS: qs Diet: DAT

LBM: 1 day ago

Discharge this AM
Dischare instructions: Office appt. 2 wks
Vicodin tab ‡ p.o. q4hr prn

PRN Medication:
Vicodin tab ‡ p.o. q4hr prn
Benadryl 25 mg p.o. hs prn q4-6hrs

Nurse's Notes

Night shift
11:00 PM Awake, oriented x3. Skin warm and dry. Pulse 88, slightly irregular, lung sounds diminished bilaterally in the lower bases. Enc. to take deep breathes, used spirometer x5. Right arm with cast, CMS-WNL. Requesting sleeping medication. Benadryl 25 mg po given. Side rails up. *S. Dolle RN*
1:30 AM Sleeping *S. Dolle RN*
4:30 AM Awake, requesting pain medication. CMS-WNL. Vicodin tab ‡ given *S. Dolle RN*
6:00 AM Resting comfortably. *S. Dolle RN*

Interactive Activity: With a partner, **use the case study and the flow charts** to:

1. Identify the pertinent patient information made known to you in the report	2. Identify the pertinent information you gathered from the flow charts	3. Review the data in columns 1 & 2 and identify information that needs follow-up

It is 7:30 AM, prioritize your plan of care for the next hour:

Time	Plan of Nursing Care

At 8:30 AM you note that Mrs. Fritz's is lethargic, very slow to respond to verbal stimuli, skin cool with slight cyanosis noted on nailbeds, P. 110 irregular, R. shallow, BP 90/70, which is lower than her usual of 130/88.

1. Identify the nursing interventions that you would plan to implement immediately	**2. Identify the nursing actions that you can delegate/assign to unlicensed personnel**

For each of the following **nursing interventions**, write an **expected patient outcome**:

1. Oxygen at 2 L/min/NP ⇨

2. Insert saline lock ⇨

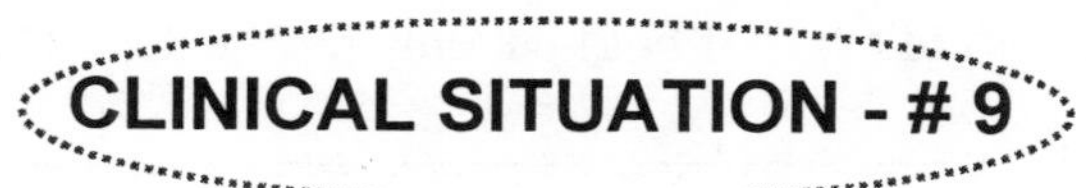

Intershift taped report at 0700:

You are assigned to the following two patients:
"Mrs. Turney is 52 yrs. old and has diabetes and hypertension. She is in for a pressure ulcer on her right heel. She is on bedrest with the right leg elevated and she only has BRP. There is a wet to dry dressing change due at 10. Her latest BP is 170/108."

"Mrs. Calderon is 73 yrs. old and was admitted with dehydration three days ago. She is eating and voiding fine. There is a possibility that she is going home today. I removed her saline lock, there was some redness at the site. She is not on any IV meds., so I decided not to restart. She says that she is going home late this afternoon, although there is no order. Her morning vital signs are 97-82-18 130/90."

Mrs. Turney's and Mrs. Calderon's **Medication Records** contain the following information:

Medication Record

Routine	Time
Glyburide 10 mg po qd	0800
Tenormin 25 po qd	1100
(patient requests these hours)	
Furosemide 20 mg po Bid	1100 - 1700
Cephalothin Sodium IVPB q6h	10-4 -10- 4

PRN Medication
MOM 30 cc prn constipation
Restoril 30 mg po HS may repeat x1

C. Turney Allergies: None

Medication Record

Routine	Time
Minipress 1 mg po qd	0900
Multivitamin tab ī po qd	0900

PRN Medication
MOM 30 cc prn constipation

M. Calderon Allergies: None

Interactive Activity: With a partner, **use the case study and the flow charts** to:

1. Identify the pertinent patient information made known to you in the <u>report</u>	2. Identify the pertinent information you gathered from the <u>flow charts</u>	3. Review the data in columns 1 & 2 and identify information that needs follow-up
Mrs. Turney:		
Mrs. Calderon:		

It is 0800, prioritize your plan of care for both patients for the next 3 hours:

Time	Plan of Nursing Care

You return from lunch at 1200 and Mrs. Turney is asking for her antihypertensive medications. You know you gave the medication, but she insists that you did not give her the meds. As you investigate, the nursing assistant tells you that Mrs. Calderon is very lethargic and unresponsive. You suddenly realize that you gave Mrs. Turney's 11:00 medications to Mrs. Calderon.

1. Identify the nursing interventions that you would plan to implement immediately	2. Make a Nurse's note entry as to how you might document this incident.

For each of the following **nursing interventions**, write an **expected patient outcome**:

1. Prepare for a code ⇨

2. Insert saline lock ⇨

CLINICAL SITUATION - # 10

Intershift taped report at 11:00 PM:

"Mrs. Jaffey, 88 yrs. old, was admitted this evening from a nursing home after the family found her lethargic and confused. Her admitting vital signs were 101 - 92 - irregular - 28 short and shallow and 110/70. Her physician was called for admitting orders, he will come in tomorrow morning to see her. She was given Tylenol at 8:30 p.m. and her current temp. is 100.6, she is still slightly confused. The family states that she had cataract surgery one week ago as an outpatient. She has an IV going. The patient in the next bed is concerned about Mrs. Jaffey's moaning."

Mrs. Jaffey's current **flow charts** contain the following information:

Nursing Care Kardex

VS q4h   Diet: DAT

LBM: On admission
IV: 0.9% NS at 75cc/hr
  #24 angio cath RFA

Lab: CBC, Chem panel, UA

PRN Medication:
Tylenol 325 mg tabs ~~ii~~ q4hrs prn temp > 101

Nurse's Notes from Skilled Nursing Facility

Documentation of latest nurse's notes:

1600 Turned, incontinent of urine, strong urine odor, incontinent pad applied. *A. Cann LVN*
1700 Family in to visit. Upset, called physician *A. Cann LVN*
1830 Transferred to hospital per order. Recent UA culture reports show + MRSA. Unable to contact physician, copy of report included with transfer. *T. Gage RN*

Interactive Activity: With a partner, **use the case study and the flow charts** to:

1. Identify the pertinent patient information made known to you in the report	2. Identify the pertinent information you gathered from the flow charts	3. Review the data in columns 1 & 2 and identify information that needs follow-up

It is 11:30 PM, prioritize your plan of care for the next hour:

Time	Plan of Nursing Care

Mrs. Jaffey is moved to a private room with isolation set up. She slept 1 - 2 hours at a time during the night and remains confused. She has developed a productive cough and is expectorating a small amount of thick creamy yellow colored phelgm. Her morning vital signs are, 100.8 - 110 - 32 - 114/82. At 6:30 AM the physician visits and leaves the following orders:

Vancomycin 500 mg q6h IVPB
Insert indwelling urinary catheter
Bedrest
Chest x-ray/ECG
Oxygen 2 L/min/NP, pulse oximeter q4hrs
I & O, enc. fluid intake

1. Identify the nursing interventions that you would plan to implement immediately	2. Identify the instructions you would give to staff and family in caring for Mrs. Jaffey

For the following **nursing intervention**, write an **expected patient outcome**:

1. Encourage fluid intake ⇨

CLINICAL SITUATION - # 11

Intershift taped report at 11:00 PM:

"Bill Rhodes, 27 yrs. old, was admitted this evening. He has been diagnosed with viral hepatitis. He is very jaundiced, his urine is very dark yellow. Intake for the shift was 100 cc and output 300 cc. He does not want to eat. He says he has not had an appetite for several days. The IV was started at 5:00 PM and is on time. His 8:00 PM vital signs are, 37.5 - 88 - 24 130/70. He is currently complaining of itching and nausea. The lab reports just arrived and I put them in the patient's chart for the physician to see in the morning."

Bill's current **flow charts** contain the following information:

Nursing Care Kardex

VS: q4hrs — Diet: DAT
Bedrest c̄ BRP

Weigh daily ☑ — I & O

IV: D5/0.9 NS @125 cc/hr
RFA # 22 g

Stool for occult blood ☐

PRN Medication:
Benadryl 50 mg capsule i q6hr prn itching
Compazine 10 mg IM q6hrs prn N/V

Current Lab Data

AST 460 units/L
ALT 800 units/L
Alk Phosphatase 200 units/L

Hgb 12.0 g/dL
Hct 36%
WBC 10,000/mm^3

BS 160 mg/dL

PT 24 secs (Pt. control 12 - 16 secs)

Total Bilirubin 14 mg/dL

Interactive Activity: With a partner, **use the case study and the flow charts** to:

1. Identify the pertinent patient information made known to you in the report	2. Identify the pertinent information you gathered from the flow charts	3. Review the data in columns 1 & 2 and identify information that needs follow-up

It is 11:30 p.m., prioritize your plan of care for the next hour:

Time	Plan of Nursing Care

→ Bill is diagnosed with Hepatitis A and is tentatively scheduled for discharge in two days.

1. Identify the discharge information that you would include in teaching Bill and his family how best to recover from Hepatitis A.

Diet: Fluids: Nausea/Vomiting: Preventing transmission:	Activity: Skin care: Sexual concerns: Alcohol intake: Follow-up care:

For the following **nursing intervention**, write the **expected patient outcome**:

1. Patient education ⇨

CLINICAL SITUATION - # 12

Intershift taped report at 7:00 AM:

"Mr. Tidwell, 67 yrs. old, has prostate cancer with metastasis to the bone. I have medicated him around the clock for pain, the last dose given at 5:00 AM. He is lethargic but responds when spoken to. He needs frequent mouth care. His urine is amber. The 6:00 AM vital signs are stable at 99 - 76 -18, 126/74. Intake is 100 cc, output is 150 cc. His wife spent the night in the room and is making arrangements for hospice care."

Mr. Tidwell's current **flow charts** contain the following information:

Nursing Care Kardex

VS: q4hrs
Bedrest

Diet: Soft

Saline lock ☑
RFA # 22 g

I & O

Urinary catheter ☑

PRN Medication:
Meperidine 100 mg q3hrs IVP prn pain

Allergies: MS
Pt: G. Tidwell

No code

Physician Progress Notes
Hosp. day #3

Assess: Skin warm, dry. T. 99
↓ oral intake
output amber urine < 600 cc/24hrs
Resp. diminished bilaterally

Alkaline phosphatase ↑
Acid phosphatase ↑

Plan: Keep comfortable
Hospice care being arranged
No code

Interactive Activity: With a partner, **use the case study and the flow charts** to:

1. Identify the pertinent patient information made known to you in the report	**2. Identify the pertinent information you gathered from the flow charts**	**3. Review the data in columns 1 & 2 and identify information that needs follow-up**

It is 7:30 AM, prioritize your plan of care for the next hour:

Time	Plan of Nursing Care

→ 2:00 PM. Mrs. Tidwell calls to inform you that Mr. Tidwell is in a lot of pain and she is very upset and tells you that the pain shots do not seem to be giving him any comfort. You call the physician and suggest an order for something stronger. The physician orders morphine sulfate 15 mg IVP q3hrs prn pain. You administer the first dose at 2:15 PM. At 2:25 PM Mrs. Tidwell calls you into the room and tells you that her husband is not breathing.

Upon assessing, you note that Mr. Tidwell has stopped breathing and there is no pulse.

1. Identify the nursing interventions that require immediate follow-up	**2. Identify and discuss the ethical issue presented in this situation.**

For the following **nursing intervention**, write the **expected outcome**:

1. Notify physician of patient's ↑ pain. ⇨

CLINICAL SITUATION - # 13

Intershift taped report at 7:00 AM:

"Mrs. Stein, 58 yrs. old, is one day postop right radical mastectomy. Her dressing is clean and dry. She has a hemovac that drained 50 cc. Her vital signs at 6:00 AM are 99.6 - 88 -24, 150/94. She is using the PCA and a new liter was hung at 6:00 AM. Her right arm is elevated on a pillow, there is some swelling and she is complaining of some numbness."

Mrs. Stein's current **flow charts** contain the following information:

Nursing Care Kardex

VS: q4hrs — Diet: Clear liquid
Up in chair — I & O

IV: Lactated Ringers @ 125 cc/hr
LFA # 18 g — Hemovac ☑

Hgb & Hct this AM ☑

Routine Medications:
Atenolol 50 mg po bid

PRN Medications:
PCA with MS at 1mg/6 min/pt. demand

History and Physical

The patient is a 58-year-old female, widow. She lives alone. Does not smoke, drinks socially. Has mild hypertension 150/94.
Meds: Atenolol 50 mg po bid
Both parents deceased - mother died of breast cancer, father died of heart disease.

Patient has two married daughters and one son.

She found a hard lump in the right breast 3 weeks ago. A biopsy was done → Stage II
CEA 5 ng/mL

Plan: Right radical mastectomy.
Chemotherapy to follow

Interactive Activity: With a partner, **use the case study and the flow charts** to:

1. Identify the pertinent patient information made known to you in the report	2. Identify the pertinent information you gathered from the flow charts	3. Review the data in columns 1 & 2 and identify information that needs follow-up

It is 7:30 AM, prioritize your plan of care for the next hour:

Time	Plan of Nursing Care

8:00 AM. You assess the following on Mrs. Stein: Alert and oriented. VS 99 - 94 - 28, 160/100. Lung sounds with fine rales in the lower bases. Surgical dressing is clean and dry. Hemovac is compressed with 10 cc reddish drainage. Right arm is elevated on a pillow. Finger puffy, c/o of a "numbness sensation." State on a 1-10 pain scale, the pain is at 2. Abdominal sounds present x4. Antiembolic hose on. Lactated Ringer's infusing, site without redness or swelling, 500 cc left.

1. Identify the nursing interventions that require immediate follow-up.	**2. Identify and discuss the postop educational needs of the patient.**

For the following **nursing intervention**, write the **expected outcome:**

1. Encourage to participate in self-care activities ⇨

CLINICAL SITUATION - # 14

Intershift taped report at 7:00 AM:

"Mr. Stockman, has left-sided heart failure. He has had a restless night with some dyspnea and a dry nonproductive cough most of the night. Crackles are heard in both lungs. He has 3+ pitting edema in both legs and sacrum. His 6:00 AM vital signs are 97.6 - 110 irregular - 34 150/100. His IV site looks slightly puffy, but there is a blood return. He just started to complain of nausea. His serum K^+ this morning is 3.0 mEq. It might be low because he is retaining fluid. His physician always come in early so I posted the results in front of the patient's chart."

Mr. Stockman's current **flow charts** contain the following information:

Nursing Care Kardex

VS: q4hrs — Diet: 2 g NA^+
↑ HOB — I & O
Bedrest with BRP
Weigh qd ☑
LBM (2 days ago)

IV: D5/0.45 NS c̄ 20 mEq KCl q12hrs
L hand # 20 g

LAB:
Digoxin level ☑
K^+, NA^+, BUN, Creatinine, AST ☑

DX: CHF — Age: 72

Medication Record

Routine	**Time**
Digoxin 0.25 mg po qd	0900
Furosemide 40 mg IVP qd	0900 - 1700
K-Dur 10 mEq po bid	0900 - 1700
Capoten 6.25 mg po tid	0900 -1700 - 2200
Colace 100 mg po qd	0900

PRN

NTG SL gr 1/150 prn chest pain

Interactive Activity: With a partner, **use the case study and the flow charts** to:

1. Identify the pertinent patient information made known to you in the report	2. Identify the pertinent information you gathered from the flow charts	3. Review the data in columns 1 & 2 and identify information that needs follow-up

It is 7:30 AM, **prioritize** your plan of care for the next hour:

Time	Plan of Nursing Care

9:00 AM. The physician has not come in to see Mr. Stockman. Mr. Stockman is alert, but experiencing increasing SOB, cough, nausea, and complaining of blurred vision. His pulse oximetry result is 88%. Pulse 116 irregular, resp. 34 short and shallow, BP 152/100. Skin cool, color with slight cyanosis. Aside from the K^+ of 3.0 mEq, Mr. Stockman's Na^+ is 135^+mEq, and his digoxin level is 2.4 ng/mL. You call the physician and learn that he is in surgery and will call you back within 30 minutes.

1. Identify the nursing interventions that require immediate follow-up.	2. Identify and discuss the postop educational needs of the patient.

For the following **nursing intervention**, write the **expected patient outcome**:

1. Lasix 40 mg IVP ⇨

CLINICAL SITUATION - # 15

Intershift taped report at 7:00 AM:

"Mrs. LaVerne, 74 yrs. old, is four days postop left hip fracture. She had a constavac that was removed yesterday. Surgical dressing is clean and dry. Pedal pulse on the left foot is present and the circulation, movement and sensation are WNL. Lung sounds with fine crackles at the lower bases in both lungs. You need to encourage her to deep breaths and use the incentive spirometer. Her 6:00 AM vital signs are 99.8 - 80 - 18, 130/82. She does not want to move, it seems like she is scared. I have medicated her two times during the night."

Mrs. LaVerne's current **flow charts** contain the following information:

Nursing Care Kardex

VS: qs Diet: Soft
HOH I & O
Ambulate with PT

LBM (2 days ago)

IV: Saline lock LFA #22g angio cath
Inserted day of surgery

Routine Medications:

Digoxin 0.125 mg po qd	9
Furosemide 10 mg po qd	9
$FeSO_4$ 300 mg po tid c̄ meals	8-12-5

PRN:

Vicodin tab i q4h prn pain

Medical History

Elderly female brought into the ED after falling at home. A fracture of the Left hip was diagnosed. She was taken to surgery and an ORIF was performed. Hgb 9.4 mg/dL, Hct 28% on admission.

She lives alone, has one son and her husband died two years ago from a cardiac condition.

Patient has a history of atrial fibrillation.

Interactive Activity: With a partner, **use the case study and the flow charts** to:

1. Identify the pertinent patient information made known to you in the report	2. Identify the pertinent information you gathered from the flow charts	3. Review the data in columns 1 & 2 and identify information that needs follow-up

It is 7:30 AM, prioritize your plan of care for the next hour:

Time	Plan of Nursing Care

You review the nurse's notes from the night shift and note the following:

12:00 PM. Alert, moaning, states leg hurts. Circulation, movement, and sensation of left leg WNL. Dressing clean and dry. Repositioned. Vicodin tab ī given for pain.
2:00 AM. Awake, states pain in leg, does not want to be touched. Left pedal pulse palpable. Repositioned.
4:00 AM. Sleeping
6:00 AM. c/o leg pain . Medicated with Vicodin tab ī.

You enter the following assessment in the nurse's notes:
7:30 AM. Awake, alert, states "did not have a good night." c/o leg pain. Left leg with pedal pulse, warm, cap. refill >2 secs. Leg elevated on pillow. Dressing clean and dry. Right leg with weak pedal pulse, swelling and redness noted at calf and thigh. Tender to touch. Lung sounds with fine crackles, encouraged to take deep breaths. Bowel sounds present x4, c/o constipation.

1. Identify the nursing interventions that require immediate follow-up.	**2. Identify the instructions that you will give the nursing assistants at this time.**

For the following **nursing intervention**, write the **expected patient outcome:**

1. Elevation of right leg ⇨

CLINICAL SITUATION - # 16

Intershift taped report at 3:00 PM:

"Mrs. Linsey was admitted with signs and symptoms of having developed a pulmonary embolism. She just had a baby two weeks ago. She has a heparin drip. The infusion pump is set at 20 cc/hr. You have 200 cc left . She slept well. Respirations are unlabored at 22. The right lower lung has diminished breath sounds. She will be started on coumadin today. She is anxious to go home and be with her baby."

Mrs. Linsey's current **flow charts** contain the following information:

Nursing Care Kardex

VS: q4hrs — Diet: Regular

Bedrest with BRP — I & O
O_2 @ 3L/min/NC prn SOB

IV: 500 cc D5W c̄ 20,000 U Heparin
LFA # 22 g angio cath
Infuse at 1000 U/hr

LAB:
Daily PTT ☑ PT in AM

Routine Medications:
Coumadin 5 mg p.o. today at 0900
Coumadin 2.5 mg p.o. today at 1700

Coagulation Record

Date	PTT	Control	Heparin dose
1st day	50 secs	25 secs	900 U/hr
2nd day	60 sec	25 secs	1000 U/hr
3rd day	90 sec	30 secs	1100 U/hr
Current	75 secs	30 secs	1000 U/hr

Interactive Activity: With a partner, **use the case study and the flow charts** to:

1. Identify the pertinent patient information made known to you in the report	2. Identify the pertinent information you gathered from the flow charts	3. Review the data in columns 1 & 2 and identify information that needs follow-up

It is 3:30 PM, prioritize your plan of care for the next hour:

Time	Plan of Nursing Care

5:00 PM. The nursing assistant informs you that the IV pump is beeping. You go into assess the pump and you notice that the heparin bag empty. You look at the infusion pump and it is set at 25 cc/hr.

1. Identify the nursing interventions that require immediate follow-up.	**2. Document your findings as you would enter them in the nursing notes.**

For the following **nursing intervention**, write the **expected patient outcome**:

1. Monitor for S & S of bleeding ⇨

CLINICAL SITUATION - # 17

Intershift taped report at 3:00 PM:

"Ms. Poe, 23 yrs. old, had an emergency appendectomy yesterday. She has Down's Syndrome. She has gotten up to the chair twice today. Surgical dressing is clean, dry, and intact. Bowel sounds are hypoactive. Her IV is infusing well, you have 200 cc left. Oral intake is 100 cc and the output is 400 cc. I have medicated her at noon for pain. Her noon vital signs are 100 - 80 - 20, 110/78."

Ms. Poe's current **flow charts** contain the following information:

Nursing Care Kardex

VS: q4hrs Diet: Clear liquid

Ambulate c̄ assistance I & O

IV: IL D5/0.9 NS @ 125 cc/hr
LFA # 22 g angio cath

Routine Medications:
Cefoxitin 2 g IVPB q6h 10-4-10-4

PRN Medications:
Meperidine 75 mg IM q4hrs prn pain c̄
Promethazine 25 mg IM q4hrs

Intake and Output Record

7 – 3 shift:

Oral:	100	Void: 8:00 AM	50
		9:00	50
		11:00	75
		12:00	50
		1:00 PM	75
IV:	900	2:00	100
IVPB:	50		
		Emesis 12:00 PM	100
Total:	1050	Total:	500

Interactive Activity: With a partner, **use the case study and the flow charts** to:

1. Identify the pertinent patient information made known to you in the report	2. Identify the pertinent information you gathered from the flow charts	3. Review the data in columns 1 & 2 and identify information that needs follow-up

It is 3:30 PM, prioritize your plan of care for the next hour:

Time	Plan of Nursing Care

8:00 PM. Ms. Poe's mother and family are at the bedside. They tell you that Ms. Poe is increasingly restless and is pulling at her surgical dressing. You note the following entries in the nursing notes:

Has voided a total of 100 cc since 4:00 PM. Emesis 100 cc greenish fluid at 6:00 PM refused dinner. Meperidine 75 mg and Promethazine 25 mg given IM at 6:00 PM.

1. Identify the nursing interventions that require immediate follow-up.	**2. Identify a rationale for each nursing intervention that you plan to implement.**

For the following **nursing intervention**, write the **expected outcome**:

1. Ambulate patient

CLINICAL SITUATION - # 18

Intershift taped report at 0700:

"Mr. Oliver has cellulitis of the right leg. He is pretty much self-care and he says he is not used to being in bed so much. He stays in a chair most of the time with his leg elevated. His I & O is fine and his vital signs are stable at 37 - 92 - 22, 164/94. He has a dry dressing on the right leg and there is no drainage. His saline lock needs to be changed today and his fingerstick bloodsugar was 110 this morning."

Mr. Oliver's current **flow charts** contain the following information:

Nursing Care Kardex

VS: q4hrs Diet: 2000 cal ADA
BRP
4x4 to right leg - Change qs
LBM 1 day ago I & O

IV: Saline lock
LFA # 22 g angio cath

Heating pad to right leg
Elevate leg on pillow
Fingerstick BS qAM 0600 ☑
C. Oliver 62 yrs. Dx: Cellulits R. Leg
Hx: Angina, Hypertension, DM Type

Medication Record

Routine:

Glyburide 10 mg po qd	0800	
Verapamil SR 240 mg po bid	0900	1700
Inderal 20 mg po bid	0900	1700
ASA 81 mg po qd	0900	
Colace 100 mg po qd	0900	

Velosef 2 gm IVPB q6hrs 2400-0600-1200-1800

PRN:
NTG SL gr 1/150 q5min x3 prn chest pain

Interactive Activity: With a partner, **use the case study and the flow charts** to:

1. Identify the pertinent patient information made known to you in the report	2. Identify the pertinent information you gathered from the flow charts	3. Review the data in columns 1 & 2 and identify information that needs follow-up

It is 0730, prioritize your plan of care for the next hour:

Time	Plan of Nursing Care

1200: Mr. Oliver returns to bed after having a BM. You note that he is SOB and his skin is cool and clammy. You assess his vital signs, his radial pulse is 110 and irregular, respirations are 32 and his BP is 170/100. He tells you that he is feeling pressure on his chest. You assist him into bed and place him in high Fowler's position.

1. Identify your follow-up nursing interventions.	**2. Identify a rationale for each nursing intervention that you plan to implement.**

For the following **nursing intervention**, write the **expected outcome**:

1. Administration of oxygen ⇨

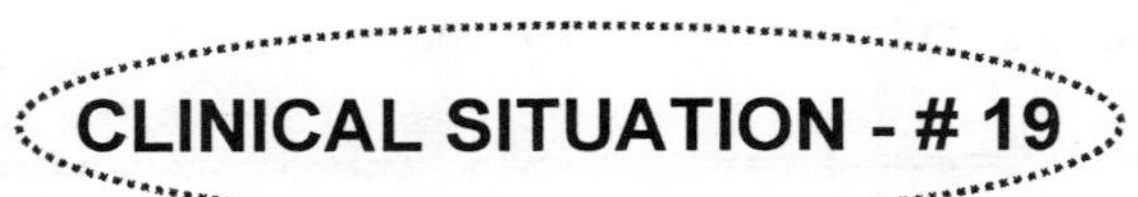

Intershift taped report at 7:00 AM:

"Mr. Isaak, 70 yrs. old, is one day postop a TURP. He has a continuous normal saline irrigation. I will hang up a new irrigation bag before I leave. He has had several clots during the shift. His vital signs are 37.2 - 90 - 22, 160/93. He is alert, cheerful, and told me that he leads a very active life. I gave him a suppository for c/o bladder spasms at 5 this morning. The IV is also very positional."

Mr. Isaak's current **flow charts** contain the following information:

Nursing Care Rand

VS q4h Diet: Clear liquids
Antiembolic hose on
LBM: On admission
IV: Lactated Ringer's at 75 cc/hr
#20 angio cath RFA

3-way indwelling cath c̄ 30 cc balloon
NS con't irrigation - keep UA free of clots

Routine Medication:
Colace 100 mg po qAM 1000
PRN Medication:
B & O supp. i q6h prn bladder spasms

Intake and Output Record

11-7 shift:

	Intake	Output
Oral:	50	1300
		(NS irrigation 1000)
IV:	300	
Total:	350	300

Interactive Activity: With a partner, **use the case study and the flow charts** to:

1. Identify the pertinent patient information made known to you in the report	2. Identify the pertinent information you gathered from the flow charts	3. Review the data in columns 1 & 2 and identify information that needs follow-up

It is 7:30 AM, prioritize your plan of care for the next hour:

Time	Plan of Nursing Care

8:00 AM: Mr. Isaak is complaining of increased pain. He is grimacing, is diaphoretic and tells you he has an urge to urinate. You note that the irrigation bag is empty and there are 50 cc of burgundy-colored urine in the urinary collection bag. There is urine leaking around the catheter.

1. Identify the nursing interventions that you would plan to implement immediately	2. Identify the follow-up nursing interventions for the rest of the shift.

For the following **nursing interventions**, write **expected patient outcomes**:

1. Bladder irrigation ⇨ [ ]

2. Enc. fluid intake ⇨ [ ]

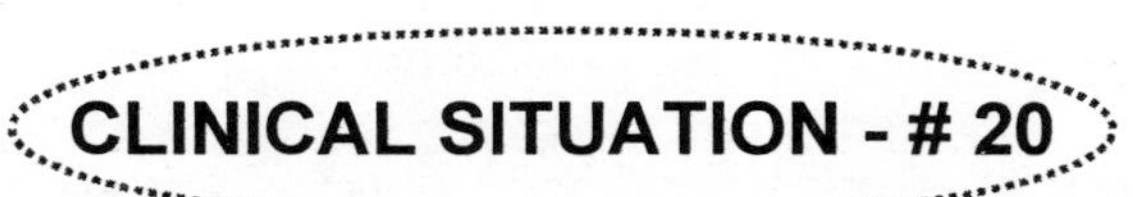

CLINICAL SITUATION - # 20

Intershift taped report at 7:00 AM:

"Mrs. Farrell, 46 yrs. old, had a TAH-BSO yesterday. She had soft bowel sounds this morning. The abdominal dressing is clean and dry. Her IV is infusing well and she has an epidural infusion with fentanyl infusing through a pump. She has not had any breakthrough pain. The epidural dressing is intact and the catheter is fine. She has been mostly on bedrest, but she is to get up to a chair this morning. The 6:00 AM vital signs are 37.5 - 78 - 18, 130/80. Her output was 500 cc."

Mrs. Farrell's current **flow charts** contain the following information:

Nursing Care Rand

VS: q4s Diet: Clear liquids
Up in chair with assistance
Incentive spirometer q1h x10 WA
LBM: Prior to admission

Urinary catheter #16 ☑

IV: D5/0.45 NS q8hrs

Routine Medication:
Fentanyl 6 cc/hr in NS via epidural catheter ordered by anesthesiologist

Intake and Output Record

Night shift:

Intake		Output	
Oral (Sips of H_2O)	50	Void	
		UA cath	500
IV:	1000		
IV (Fentanyl)	48		

Interactive Activity: With a partner, **use the case study and the flow charts** to:

1. Identify the pertinent patient information made known to you in the report	2. Identify the pertinent information you gathered from the flow charts	3. Review the data in columns 1 & 2 and identify information that needs follow-up

It is 7:30 AM, prioritize your plan of care for the next hour:

Time	Plan of Nursing Care

At 8:30 AM. Mrs. Farrell gets up with assistance to sit in a chair. As she walks slowly to the chair, she steps on some of the tubings. The nursing assistance tells you that the infusion pump is beeping. You go into assess and note that the epidural infusion pump it beeping and the patient's epidural dressing is pulled from the patient's back. The epidural catheter seems to be pulled out.

1. Identify the nursing interventions that you would plan to implement immediately	2. Document your findings as you would enter them in a nursing notes.

For each of the following **nursing intervention**, write an **expected patient outcome**:

1. Cover epidural site with 4x4 ⇨

SECTION FOUR

Answer Keys

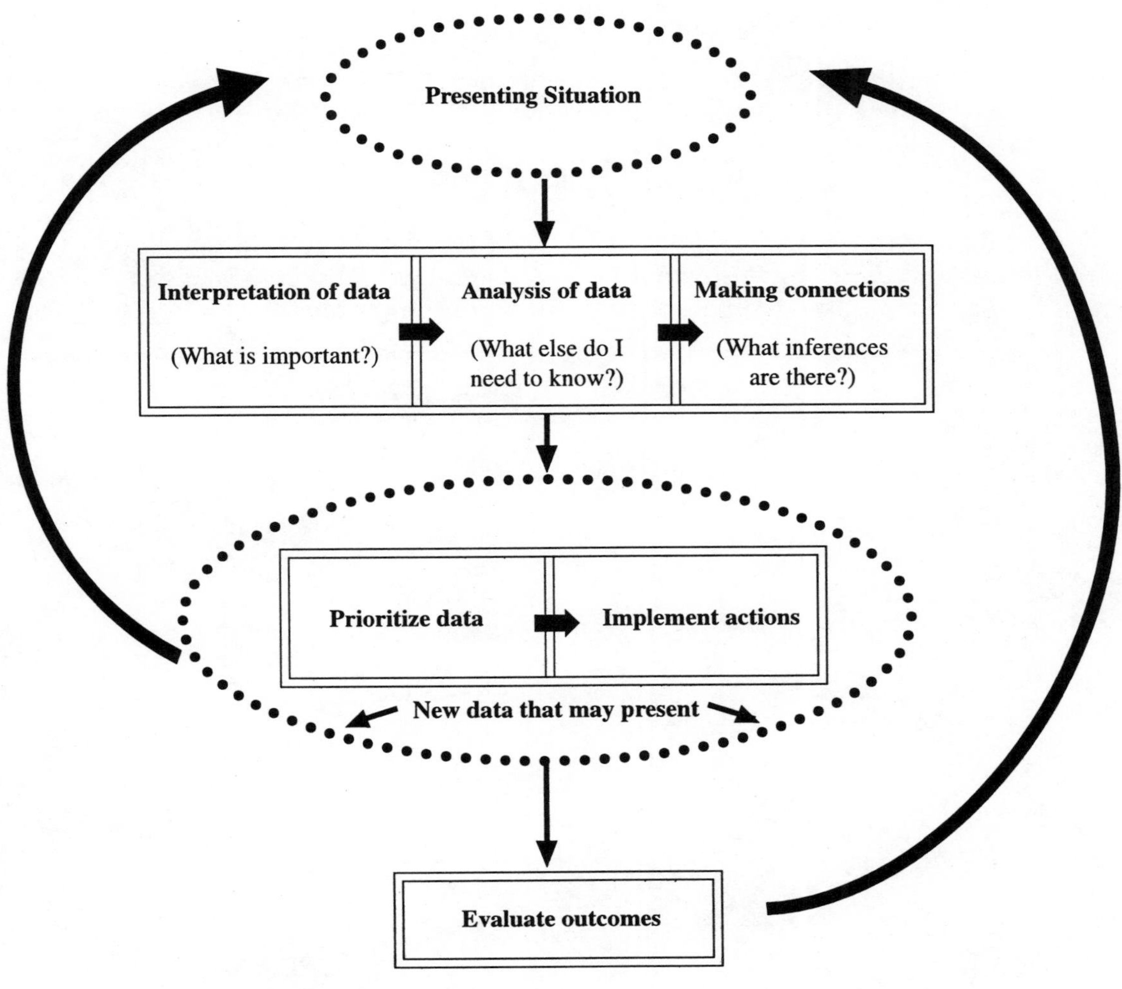

VITAL SIGNS

List the routes for taking a **temperature**:

1. Oral
2. Axillary
3. Rectal
4. Tympanic

Use the diagram to identify the **pulse sites** in the body.

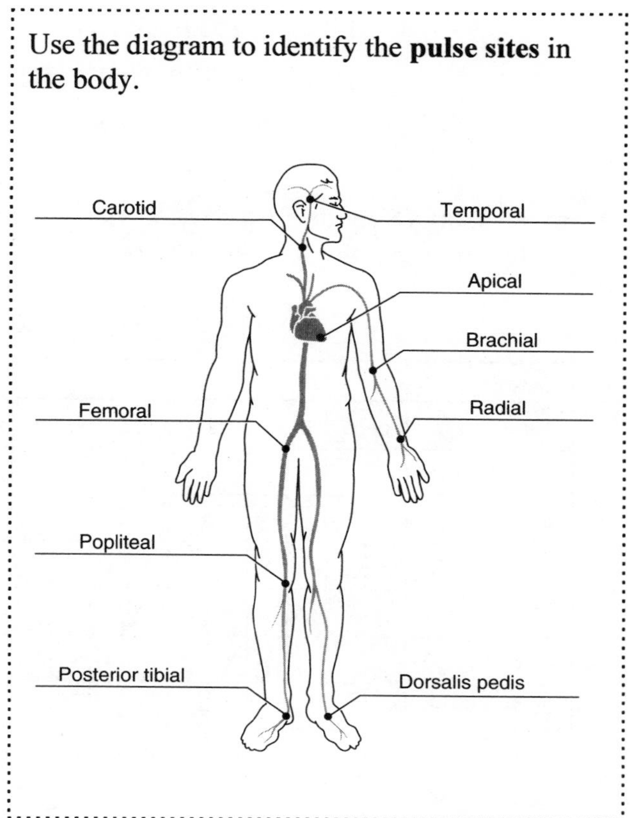

The **blood pressure** may be auscultated in the antecubital & popliteal space.

Case Study: Stanley Moore has been having a high fever for 2 days. After visiting the physician's office, he was found to be febrile. Additionally, Mr. Moore is complaining of chills, night sweats, anorexia and fatigue. He is admitted to the hospital. The physician's orders include vital signs every four hours. On admission he was experiencing pyrexia. His admission vital signs are T 102.4°F – P 96 – R 26 – BP 148/88.

Pertinent Terminology	Definition
Vital signs	The body temperature, pulse, respiration, and blood pressure.
Temperature	The degree of heat in the body measured in degrees.
Pulse	The wave of blood pumped into the arterial wall with each heartbeat.
Respiration	The process of breathing; involves the exchange of O_2 and CO_2.
Blood pressure	The pressure exerted against the arterial walls with the heartbeat.
Febrile	Fever; the body temperature above the normal range.
Pyrexia	Increase in the body temperature; fever.
Anorexia	Diminished, loss, or lack of appetite.
Fatigue	Tiredness; exhaustion.

From the case study, record today's date and the 0800 admission vital signs (VS) on the **Graphic Sheet** below. Enter the following vital signs for today:

1200 T 103.6 – P 108 – R 32 – BP 160/76

1600 T 101.2 – P 98 – R 28 – BP 154/82

2000 T 100.0 – P 80 – R 24 – BP 150/90

Record the 0800 VS for the next day: T 99.6 – P 72 – R 18 – BP 146/94

Draw a line between the temperature recordings to create a graph.

GRAPHIC SHEET

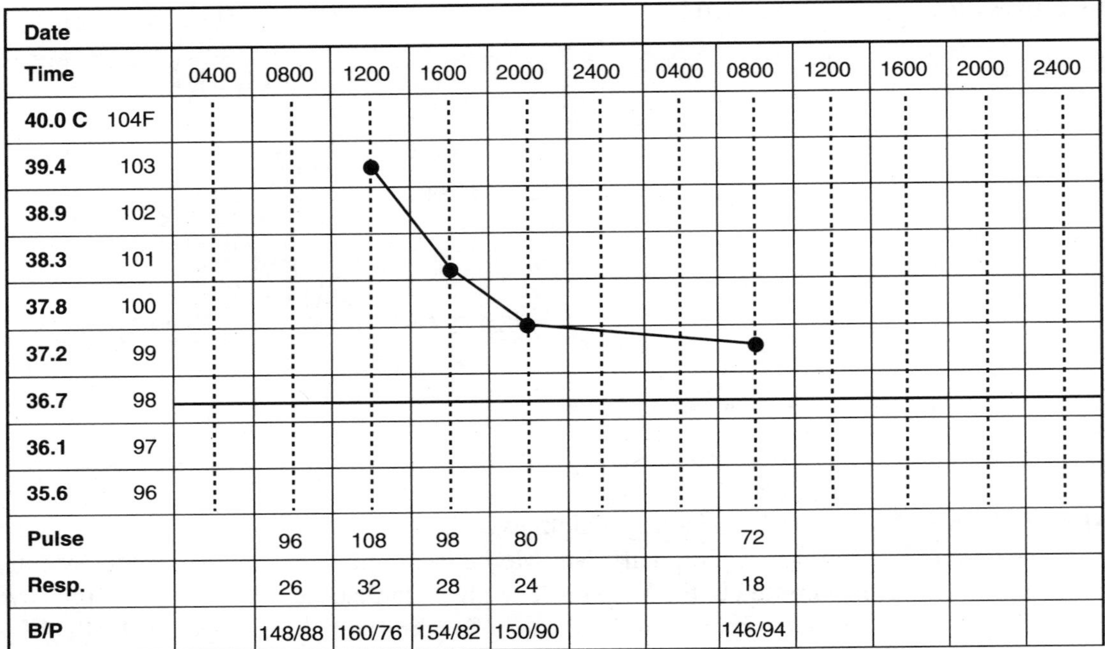

Date												
Time	0400	0800	1200	1600	2000	2400	0400	0800	1200	1600	2000	2400
40.0 C 104F												
39.4 103												
38.9 102												
38.3 101												
37.8 100												
37.2 99												
36.7 98												
36.1 97												
35.6 96												
Pulse		96	108	98	80			72				
Resp.		26	32	28	24			18				
B/P		148/88	160/76	154/82	150/90			146/94				

Interactive Activity: With a partner, identify the **normal range(s)** for the vital signs in the adult.

Body temperature
- **Oral** 98.6°F or 37°C
- **Axillary** 97.6°F or 36.5°C
- **Rectal** 99.5°F or 37.5°C

Pulse 60 – 100 bpm

Respirations 12 – 20

Blood Pressure 120/80

BLOOD PRESSURE

The average **blood pressure** for an adult is 120/80 mm Hg.

Factors that affect the **blood pressure** include:

1. Age
2. Sex
3. Exercise
4. Stress
5. Race
6. Obesity
7. Medications
8. Cardiac disease
9. Diurnal variation
10. Cigarette smoking

Identify the parts of the following items used in obtaining a blood pressure:

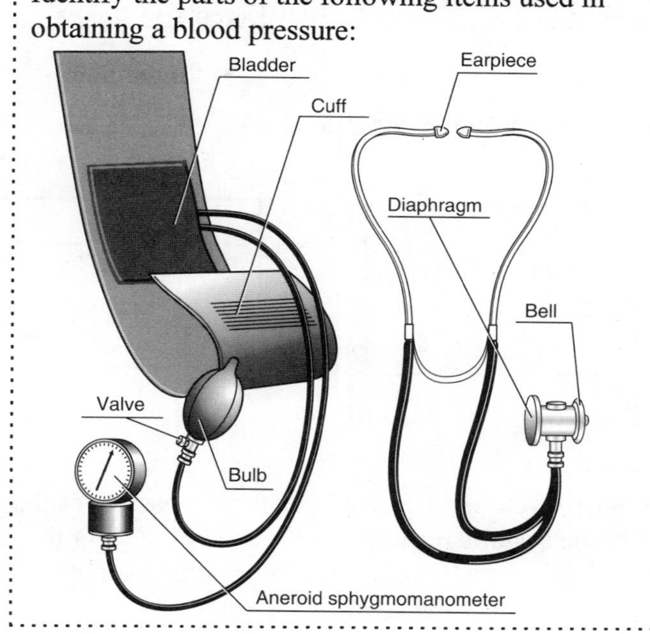

Case Study: Mr. Harold is a 65 yr. old African-American man. He goes weekly to the Hypertension Clinic for blood pressure checks. He has a 20-year history of smoking 2 packs of cigarettes a day. His father died from heart disease and his brother also has hypertension. His current blood pressure (BP) reading is 174/104 and he is complaining of a headache and dizziness when getting up in the morning.

Pertinent Terminology	Definition
Blood pressure	Pressure exerted against the arterial walls by the heartbeat.
Systolic pressure	Pressure exerted against the arterial walls by the heart during contraction.
Diastolic pressure	Least amount of pressure on the arterial walls occurring during heart relaxation.
Korotkoff's sounds	The sounds heard during ausculation of the blood pressure.
Pulse pressure	The difference between the systolic and diastolic pressure.
Hypertension	Systolic pressure >140 mm Hg and diastolic >90 mm Hg.
Hypotension	Systolic pressure <100 mm Hg.
Orthostatic hypotension	Lowering of BP when changing from a horizontal to vertical position.
Auscultatory gap	Temporary absence of the Korotkoff's sound.

From the case study, identify the **factors** that predisposed Mr. Harold for developing hypertension:

Race	Age	Cigarette smoking
Lifestyle	Heredity	Gender

§ The clinic nurse monitors Mr. Harold's blood pressure for three days:

Day I	
11:00 am	210/110
11:15 am	202/104
11:30 am	190/98

Day 2	
11:00 am	188/100
11:15 am	170/98
11:30 am	164/94

Day 3	**11:00 am**
Lying	178/100
Sitting	166/90
Standing	150/90

Interactive Activity: Record the blood pressure readings on the flow sheet using the symbol "V" to identify the systolic reading and the symbol "Λ" for the diastolic reading. Connect both symbols with a straight line. Identify the orthostatic blood pressure readings with the appropriate symbols. Compare your flow sheet with a partner.

BLOOD PRESSURE FLOW SHEET

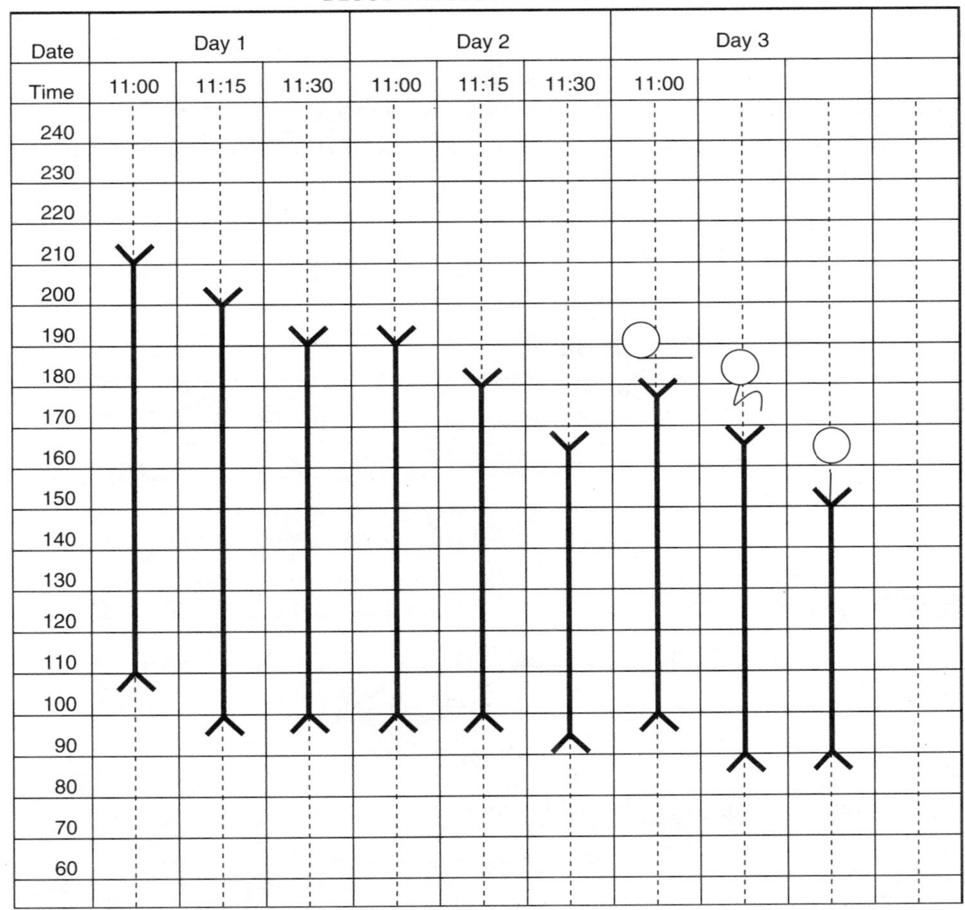

INFECTION CONTROL/TRANSMISSION OF ORGANISMS

Provide examples of the following elements found in the **chain of infection**:

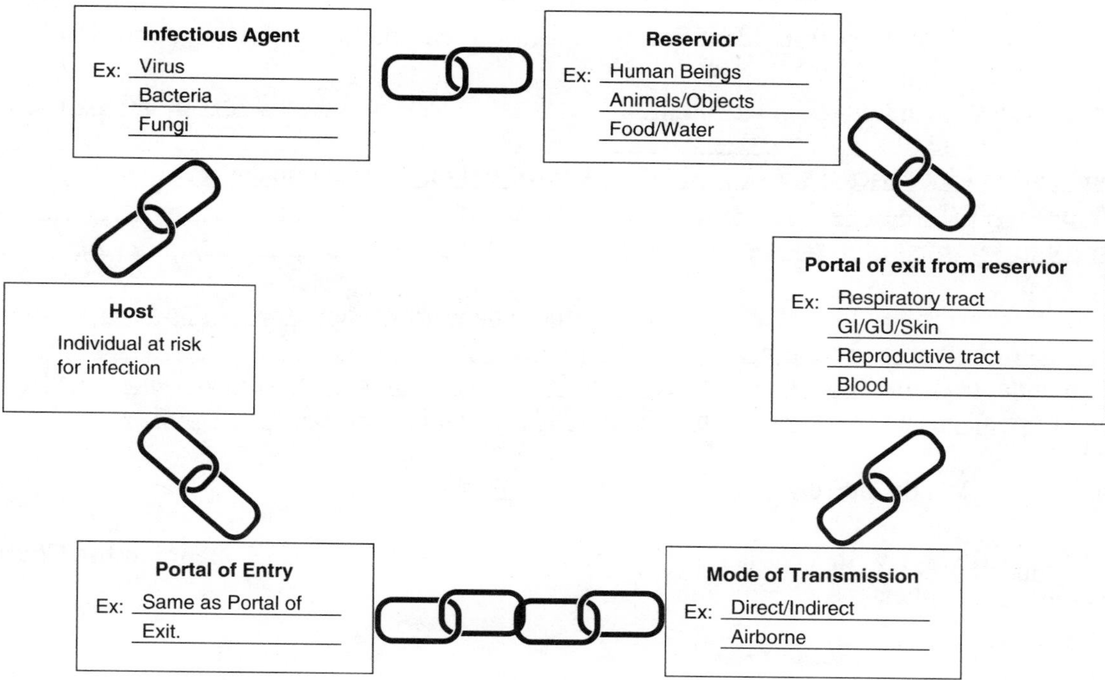

Case Study: Keli has recently begun nursing school. During her second week in the clinical setting, Keli takes care of Mr. Wu, a 79-yr.-old patient, who was admitted with dehydration. He has a recent history of shingles that is in the convalescent stage of illness. Mr. Wu's skin is very dry, his oral temperature is 100.4°F. His urine is very dark amber and his WBC is 13,000 mm³.

Pertinent Terminology	Definition
Shingles	Herpes zoster.
Dehydration	Loss of water from the body.
Incubation stage	Time between entry of organism and appearance of clinical symptoms .
Prodromal stage	Onset of nonspecific symptoms (ie, flu-like) to more specific symptoms.
Illness stage	Manifestation of signs and symptoms of the disease.
Convalescent stage	Recovery phase, symptoms disappear.
Asepsis	Freedom from infection. The absence of pathogenic organisms.
Nosocomial	Hospital-acquired infections.

From the case study, identify the **factors** that make Mr. Wu susceptible for getting an infection?

Dehydration — Age

History of recent shingles — Increased WBC

Explain **why** each of the **factors** identified make Mr. Wu susceptible to getting an infection.

1. **Age** - The normal age-related physiological changes increase the susceptibility of elderly patients to become ill.
2. **Dehydration** - increases the risk of skin breakdown and electrolyte imbalance.
3. **Increased WBC** - body's defenses are compromised with current illness.
4. **History of recent shingles** - compromised immune system.

Define **medical asepsis**: Medical asepsis refers to those measures taken to reduce and control the transmission of microorganisms (handwashing, gloving, gowning, etc.).

Define **surgical asepsis**: Surgical asepsis refers to those measures that keep objects and areas free from microorganisms and prevent the introduction of pathogens to the patient.

In caring for Mr. Wu the nurse will use **medical** asepsis.

Interactive Activity: With a partner, fill in the **diagrams** with the proper **elements in the Chain of Infection** as it applies to each situation:

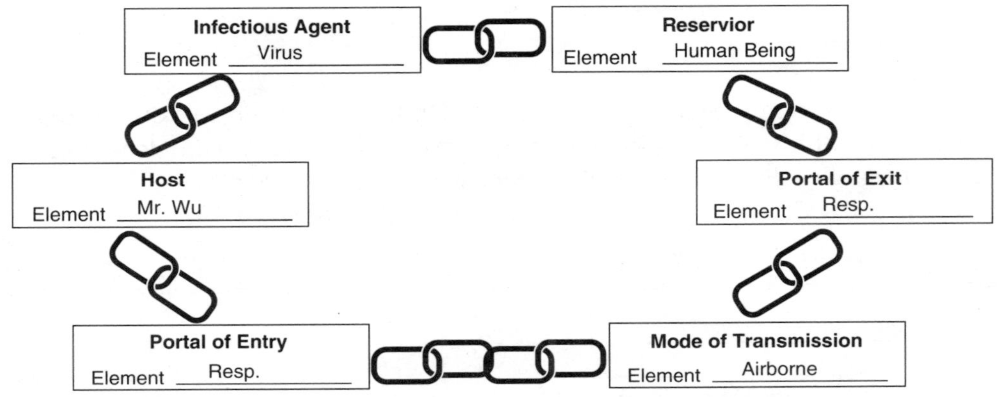

2. A nursing assistant goes from patient to patient without changing gloves.

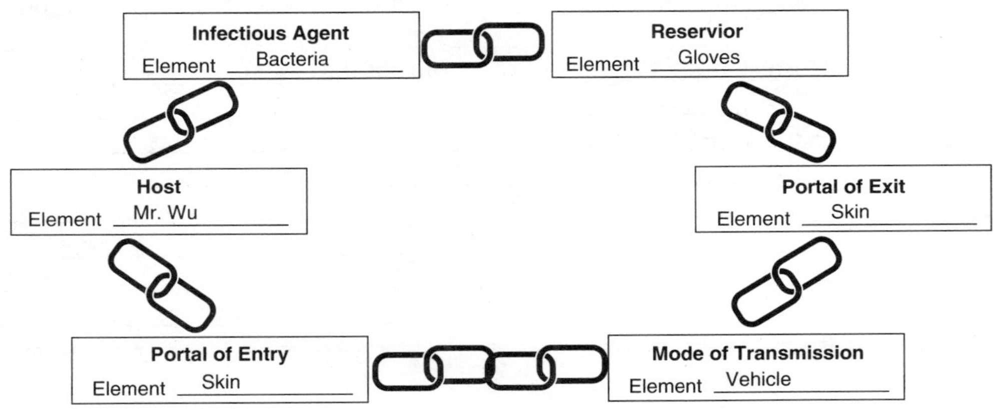

INTRODUCTION TO THE ASSESSMENT PROCESS

List the **methods** available to the nurse for the **collection of patient data**:

1. Interview
2. Observation
3. Physical assessment
4. Patient's chart

List the **parts of the Patient's Chart** that assist the nurse in the **collection of patient data**:

1. History and physical record
2. Nurses notes
3. Admission data
4. M.D. progress notes
5. Lab/Diagnostic studies
6. Rehab/PT/OT/Other services notes

Draw a line to connect all the **Objective Data**.

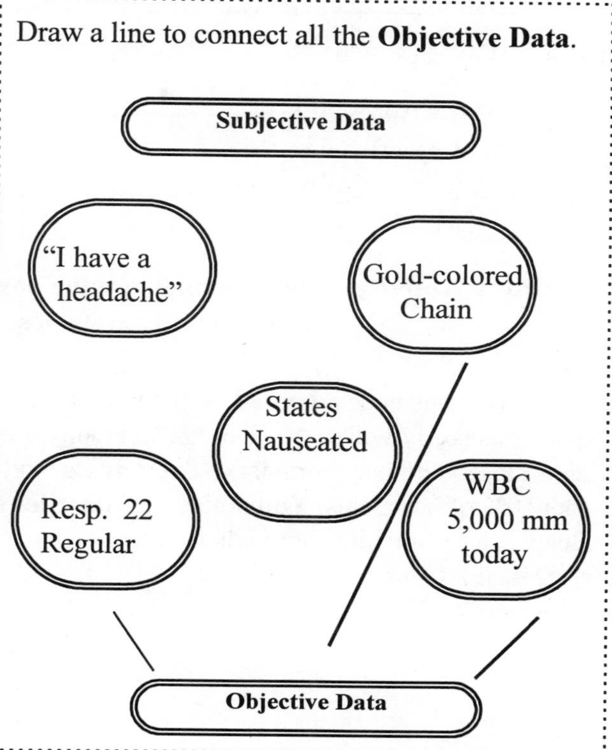

Case Study: Mrs. Clark has been admitted to the hospital for the birth of her baby. Her husband is by her side. You observe that she is very pleasant but cries out with each contraction. She tells you "I feel a lot of pressure in my back." Her chart indicates that she is 26 yrs. old and that she has a 6-yr.-old son.

Pertinent Terminology	Definition
Assessment	The collection, verification, organization and communication of subjective and objective data.
Subjective data	Information perceived by the patient—covert data.
Objective data	Data observed by the nurse—overt data.
Clustering data	Organizing pertinent subjective and objective data together to provide meaningful information.
Validation of data	The review and verification of data to ensure that data are factual and accurate.
Primary source	Regarding information, the patient is the primary person who can give information about his/her health issues.
Secondary source	Other sources who can provide data regarding the patient, such as family members, the patient's chart, support persons, and health professionals.

Use the case study to identify the following information:

	Source (Primary/Secondary)
✎ List the **objective data**:	
1. Admitted to hospital; husband at bedside	
2. Cries out with contractions	Primary
3. Age 26	Secondary
4. Has a 6-year-old son	Secondary
✎ List the **subjective data**:	
1. "I feel a lot of pressure on my back."	Primary

Interactive Activity: With a partner, **use the box to identify subjective and objective data** from the case studies:

§ Mrs. Toby has been admitted with depression. She answers questions softly with a "yes" or "no" response. She wants her door closed and her room dark. She refuses visitors and only eats 10% of her meals. You notice that she cries regularly and sleeps a lot. She bites her nails frequently.

> Objective data
>
> § Answers questions softly.
> § Door closed/dark room.
> § Refuses visitors.
> § Eats 10% of meals.
> § Cries regularly.
> § Sleeps a lot.
> § Bites nails frequently.
>
> Subjective data
>
> NONE

§ Mr. Peale had surgery one day ago. He tells you that he has been very independent all his life and hates being sick. He has refused his pain medication all morning. You notice that he refuses to get out of bed, he moans quietly every now and then, he is sweaty and his hands are clenched tightly. His surgical dressing is clean and he says everything is fine when you ask him a question.

> Objective data
>
> § Surgery one day ago.
> § Refused pain medication.
> § Refused to get out of bed.
> § Moans every now and then.
> § He is sweaty.
> § Hands clenched tightly.
>
> Subjective data
>
> § Independent/hates being sick.
> § Says everything is fine.

§ Mr. Keil informs the nursing assistant that he is nauseated. He has refused his lunch. You go in to check him and you notice 100 cc of clear yellow emesis. He tells you that he vomited. His wife is at his bedside.

> Objective data
>
> § Refused his lunch.
> § Emesis 100 cc.
> § Wife at bedside.
>
> Subjective data
>
> § CNA stated pt. nauseated.
> § He says he vomited.

INTRODUCTION TO FORMULATING A NURSING DIAGNOSIS

List the **5 steps of the Nursing Process**:

1. Assessment
2. Diagnosis (problem identification)
3. Planning
4. Implementation
5. Evaluation

Circle the **words** that may be used to give specific meaning to the Nursing Diagnosis statement:

Related to

(Increased) Well

(Altered)

High Risk

(Acute)

(Impaired)

Sign/Symptom

Due to Possible

The **NANDA Nursing Diagnoses** are classified and formulated to address the patient's health problems which can be:

1. Actual
2. Potential/Risk for/High Risk
3. Possible
4. Wellness

Case Study: Judy, the home health nurse makes the following observations and documents the following after visiting Mr. Toby: Mr. Toby lives alone, his only son lives 60 miles away, visits monthly and calls weekly. Mr. Toby stays indoors all day. His vision is poor and he is not able to drive.

Pertinent Terminology	Definition
NANDA	North American Nursing Diagnosis Association.
Nursing Process	A method of problem solving that includes patient participation.
Assessment	The first step of the nursing process and includes the collection, verification, organization, and communication of data.
Nursing Diagnosis	The second step of the nursing process that involves the formulation of the diagnostic statement.
Defining Characteristics	The subjective and objective data that support the identified nursing diagnosis.
Planning	The third step of the nursing process that involves the identification of measureable, realistic outcomes and goals.
Implementation	The fourth step of the nursing process which involves the implementation of the plan of care.
Evaluation	The final step of the nursing process which involves assessing, judging, and evaluating the extent to which the outcomes and goals were met.
Etiology	The contributing factor used in the nursing diagnostic statement to identify patient health needs that assist in the formulation of the nursing diagnosis.

From the case study, **check off (✓) the Nursing Diagnosis** most appropriate for Mr. Toby (✳ Use a Nursing Diagnosis book to validate your selection):

Nursing Diagnoses:

- ____ Ineffective coping
- _✓_ Risk for loneliness
- ____ Social isolation

List the **defining characteristics** for the **nursing diagnosis** you selected:

✳ Lives alone ✳ Stays indoors ✳ Poor vision

✳ Son lives 60 miles away ✳ Unable to drive

☞ **Further documentation** by the home health nurse states: Mr. Toby has lost 10 lbs. since the last visit—two weeks ago. He now is malnourished. Mr. Toby is on a limited income. He needs the services of a nutritionist and a community service that delivers meals to homebound individuals.

From the **further documentation** data, **check off (✓) the Nursing Diagnosis** most appropriate for Mr. Toby:

Nursing Diagnoses:

- ____ Social isolation
- ____ Knowledge deficit
- _✓_ Altered nutrition: less than body requirements

List the **current pertinent defining characteristics** for the nursing diagnosis you selected:

✳ limited income ✳ lost 10 lbs in two weeks ✳ malnourished

Interactive Activity: With a partner, review the following case studies and **identify** the **defining characteristics** that relate to the **Nursing Diagnosis** written next to each situation:

Case Study	✳ Defining Characteristics
Mrs. Shaw has a Stage II pressure ulcer on her right heel. She has been on bedrest and her right leg is elevated.	Impaired skin integrity: actual ✳Immobility/disruption of skin layers
Mr. Clarke has oral lesions in his mouth caused by a treatment of chemotherapy. He complains of pain and his mouth is red.	Altered oral mucous membranes ✳Oral lesions, pain, redness, chemotherapy
Mrs. Morning-Star is scheduled for surgery in the morning. She says that she is very scared because her grandmother died having surgery.	Fear ✳States fear

ASSESSMENT OF THE ELDERLY PATIENT

List the **interventions** that would assist in communicating with an elderly patient who is experiencing hearing loss related to the aging process:

1. Speak facing patient, in close proximity
2. Lower pitch of voice
3. Speak clearly, articulate well
4. Use short sentences
5. Use nonverbal communication if necessary

List the **interventions** that would assist in an elderly patient who is experiencing vision problems related to the aging process:

1. Avoid or reduce glare
2. Use night-light/ensure adequate lighting
3. Use contrasting colors (avoid green/blue)
4. Color code edges of steps
5. Face patient when speaking

Mark an **"X"** in the appropriate column that identifies the effects of aging on the following:

	Decreased	**Increased**
Sensory perception	☒	☐
Visual acuity	☒	☐
Gag reflex	☒	☐
Skin tissue elasticity	☒	☐
Body temperature	☒	☐
Cardiac output	☒	☐
RBC production	☒	☐
Plasma viscosity	☐	☒
Lung capacity	☒	☐
Residual urine	☐	☒

Case Study: The following information was given to a group of students regarding the assessment of an elderly patient: Responds slowly, but appropriately to all questions, skin warm, dry, thin and flakey. Skin turgor >3 secs. Capillary refill >3 secs. Respirations short and shallow, lung sounds with bilateral crackles. 50% intake, states food is very bland. BM this morning moderate amount formed hard stool. Bilateral lower extremities with 1+ pitting edema. Toenails yellowish, thick. Vital signs T 99°F – P 84 – R 16 – BP 160/80.

Pertinent Terminology	**Definition**
Arcus senilis	The opaque whitish ring that partially or fully encircles the outer margin of the iris.
Edema	Increased accumulation of fluid in the interstitial spaces.
Pitting edema	The development of an indentation or pit on edematous tissue when depressed. The degree of pitting is measured by a scale (1+, 2+, 3+, and 4+).
Kyphosis	Excessive curvature of the spine, humpback.
Presbycusis	The progressive loss of hearing acuity and auditory ability to discriminate speech frequencies and high-pitched sounds.
Presbyopia	The decline in the ability of the eyes to accommodate to close work.
Turgor	The elasticity or resiliency of the skin. Factors such as dehydration and the aging process affect skin elasticity.

Use the information from the case study below to mark an "**X**" on the data that are representative of the normal effects of the aging process:

- **X** Responds slowly, but appropriately to all questions
- **X** Skin warm, dry, thin, and flakey
- **X** Skin turgor >3 secs. Capillary refill >3 secs
- ____ Respirations short and shallow, lung sounds with bilateral crackles
- **X** 50% intake, states food is very bland
- ____ BM this morning formed hard stool
- ____ Bilateral lower extremities with 1+ pitting edema.
- **X** Toenails yellowish, thick
- ____ Vital signs T 99°F – P 84 – R 16 – BP 160/80

Interactive Activity: With a partner, use the information provided to **(1) <u>underline</u>** the assessment data that represent the **effects of the normal aging process** and **(2) select** the NANDA Nursing Diagnosis most appropriate for the situation:

ASSESSMENT DATA	NURSING DIAGNOSIS
Wife in to see patient, states that husband is confused this morning, does not know that he is in the hospital. Further patient assessment, PERRL, <u>whitish ring noted around the margins of the iris</u>, <u>uses glasses</u>. Mouth dry, wears upper dentures.	☐ Altered thought processes ☐ Knowledge deficit ☒ Acute confusion ☐ Impaired memory
<u>Skin pale, translucent</u>. <u>Lower extremities thin, pedal pulses weak, palpable</u>. States has <u>loss of a small amount of urine when coughs</u>. Shortness of breath, R 28, mouth breathing. <u>Abdomen round</u>, soft, nontender. <u>Temp. 96.8</u>.	☐ Functional incontinence ☐ Hypothermia ☐ Altered peripheral tissue perfusion ☒ Ineffective breathing pattern
Transfers independently out of bed, complained of dizziness when coming to a standing position, gait slow. <u>Anterior-posterior diameter of chest increased</u>. Soft diet, intake 70%.	☐ Impaired physical mobility ☒ Risk for injury ☐ Altered health maintenance ☐ Altered nutrition, less than body requirements

THE PATIENT WITH FLUID & ELECTROLYTE IMBALANCE

List the **adult normal values** for the following electrolytes:

1. Sodium (Na^+) = 136 - 145 mEq/L
2. Potassium (K^+) = 3.5 - 5.0 mEq/L
3. Chloride (Cl^-) = 96 - 106 mEq/L
4. Calcium (Ca^{2+}) = 9.0 - 11.0 mg/dL
5. Phosphate (PO_4^-) = 3.0 - 4.5 mg/dL
6. Magnesium (Mg^{2+}) = 1.8 - 3.0 mg/dL

Write in the appropriate medical terminology for the serum laboratory values below:

Mg^{2+} 3.5 mg/dL	=	Hypermagnesemia
K^+ 2.5 mEq/L	=	Hypokalemia
Cl^- 90 mEq/L	=	Hypochloremia
Na^+ 132 mEq/L	=	Hyponatremia
Ca^{2+} 8.5 mg/dL	=	Hypocalcemia
PO_4^- 5.1 mg/dL	=	Hyperphosphatemia

Case Study: Mr. Howard, 36 yrs. old, was admitted with gastroenteritis. He has been vomiting and having severe diarrhea for two days. He is very weak. The current lab results are: Na^+ 128 mEq/L, K^+ 2.8 mEq/L, Cl^- 90 mEq/L. The physician orders: IV of 0.9% NS at 100 cc/hr, NPO and I & O.

Pertinent Terminology	Definition
Sodium (Na^+)	Primary extracellular cation. Maintains osmotic pressure. Changes affect water balance since water follows salt.
Potassium (K^+)	Primary intracellular cation. Affects most body systems. Vital for normal neuromuscular and cardiac functions.
Chloride (Cl^-)	Major negative ion in the extracellular fluid. Closely linked with sodium. Helps to maintain osmotic pressure in the serum.
Calcium (Ca^{2+})	Found in free or ionized state and bound to plasma proteins. Helps in skeletal formation, neuromuscular activity, and blood coagulation.
Phosphate (PO_4^-)	Major intracellular anion. Closely linked with calcium. Promotes neuromuscular activity, cell division, and metabolism of foods.
Magnesium (Mg^{2+})	Mostly an intracellular ion. Essential for neuromuscular and the enzyme functions of the cell.
Third space syndrome	A fluid shift into the interstitial spaces that remains trapped in these spaces. Common sites include the abd., the pleural and peritoneal cavity, and the pericardial sac.
Edema	Fluid retention in the interstitial spaces. Common sites are the sacrum and lower extremities. Most often indicative of impaired venous return.
Pitting edema	The presence of edema in the tissue which remains pitted or indented when pressed.

From the case study, identify the abnormal laboratory results. List the **major clinical signs or symptoms** that you would assess with each abnormal value:

* Na^+ 128 mEq/L = Apprehension, lethargy, confusion, abdominal cramps, weak, thready pulse, orthostatic hypotension, dry skin (etc.).

* Cl^- 90 mEq/L = Clinical signs and symptoms similar to Na^+ imbalance.

* K^+ 2.8 mEq/L = Anorexia, vomiting, constipation, distention, ileus, muscle weakness, cramps, dysrhythmias, weak pulse, shallow respirations, confusion, (etc.).

☞ **Follow-up case study**: Mr. Howard's vomiting and diarrhea has begun to subside in the evening and the M.D. has ordered a clear liquid diet. Mr. Howard's **24 hour Intake and Output** for the day is charted below:

24 Hour Intake/Output Record

Intake		Output	
IV =	2400	Emesis =	950
Oral =	120	Diarrhea =	900
		Urine =	750
	2520 cc		2600 cc

☞ Based on the case study and Intake and Output Record **select** the most appropriate **NANDA Nursing Diagnoses** for Mr. Howard:

___ Fluid volume excess
_X_ Diarrhea
_X_ Altered nutrition: Less than body requirements
_X_ Fluid volume deficit
_X_ Impaired skin integrity
_X_ Risk for injury

Interactive Activity: With a partner, read the case study below and write a **rationale** for each of the nursing interventions listed:

Case Study	Nursing Interventions	Rationale
Sallie May was admitted with heart failure. The nursing diagnosis of "Fluid volume excess r/t noncompliance to dietary Na+ restriction" is listed in her NCP. Digoxin 0.25 mg qd po, Furosemide 40 mg qd po, and K-dur 10 mEq po tid are her medications.	▸ Weigh daily	Assess fluid loss/gain
	▸ Monitor I & O	Assess fluid loss/gain
	▸ Take apical pulse	✓for electrolyte imbalance
	▸ Assess skin	✓skin integrity
	▸ Assess lungs	✓for adventitious sounds
	▸ ✓ Neck veins	✓for ECF overload

GENERAL NUTRITION

List the **four therapeutic diets** commonly encountered in the clinical setting (exclude the special diets):

1. Regular diet
2. Soft diet
3. Full liquid diet
4. Clear liquid diet

List the most common methods of providing enteral nutrition:

1. Orally
2. Nasogastric tube feeding
3. Gastrostomy tube feeding
4. Jejunostomy tube feeding

Draw a line to connect the following **foods** with the appropriate **common therapeutic diets** encountered in the clinical setting:

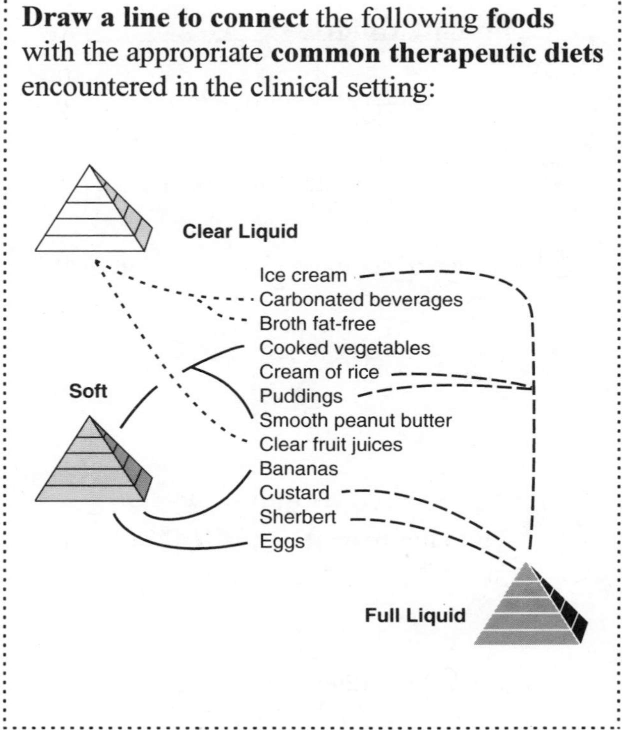

Case Study: Mr. Grier, 68 yrs. old, had a Cerebral Vascular Accident (CVA) two weeks ago. He has right-sided hemiplegia. The nursing care rand indicates that Mr. Grier is on a soft, pureed diet and is on Intake and Output.

Pertinent Terminology	Definition
Regular diet	The standard diet consisting of appropriate servings and foods from all the food groups.
Soft diet	Consists of foods that are easily chewed and digested, low in fiber and fat.
Full liquid	Consists of foods that are liquid or that liquify at room temperature. Low in iron, protein and calories.
Clear liquid	Consists of tea, coffee, clear broths, and carbonated beverages. Nutritionally and calorically inadequate.
Enteral nutrition	Nutrition provided through the gastrointestinal tract, includes oral and tube feedings.
Gastric lavage	Feeding into the stomach with a small tube passed through the nares, pharynx, and esphagus into the stomach—a nasogastric tube.
Gastrostomy tube	The insertion of a catheter through an opening into the stomach for feeding purposes.
PEG	Percutaneous endoscopic gastrostomy—procedure for the insertion of a gastric tube for feeding the patient.
Jejunostomy tube	The insertion of a catheter through an opening into the jejunum.

Use the information from the case study to **mark an "X"** on the most appropriate feeding guidelines for Mr. Grier who has right-sided hemiplegia:

Feeding Guidelines

- ☐ Give water frequently with the food
- ☒ Check right cheek for "pocketing"
- ☐ Place in semi-Fowler's position
- ☒ Allow family to feed Mr. Grier
- ☒ Place in high Fowler's position
- ☒ Give thickened juices
- ☒ Provide finger foods
- ☐ Lie flat after feeding

Interactive Activity: With a partner, use the case studies related to Mr. Grier. For each situation **prioritize the NANDA Nursing Diagnosis**, **#1** = Highest priority, **#2** = Important, and **#3** = Need to monitor.

Case Study	NANDA Nursing Diagnosis
Mr. Grier's intake for last 24 hrs = 1250 cc and his output = 725 cc. He is fatigued and needs to be reminded to drink and eat. His skin is dry and flaky. Skin turgor-tenting. Oral mucous membranes dry, teeth missing. Urine color is dark yellow.	__1__ Fluid volume deficit r/t decreased fluid intake secondary to fatigue __3__ Risk for altered oral mucous membranes r/t insufficient intake of fluids __2__ Risk for impaired skin integrity r/t dry, thin skin secondary to aging
Mr. Grier began to cough forcefully while being fed. The feeding was stopped and the M.D. ordered for him to be NPO. Mr. Grier has lost 3 lbs in one week. He has an IV of D_5W infusing at 75 cc/hr. It is difficult to get him out of bed, since he is weak and does not assist in the transfer.	__2__ Altered nutrition r/t weakness, fatigue and NPO status __1__ Risk for aspiration r/t impaired swallowing __3__ Risk for impaired skin integrity r/t prolonged bedrest

COMPLICATIONS OF DIABETES MELLITUS

List the **causes** that precipitate **hypoglycemic reactions**:

» Incorrect insulin dose
» Delaying or skipping a meal
» Alcohol consumption
» Increased physical exercise
» Drug interactions

For each line identify a specific **long-term complication**, i.e., stroke, associated with Diabetes Mellitus.

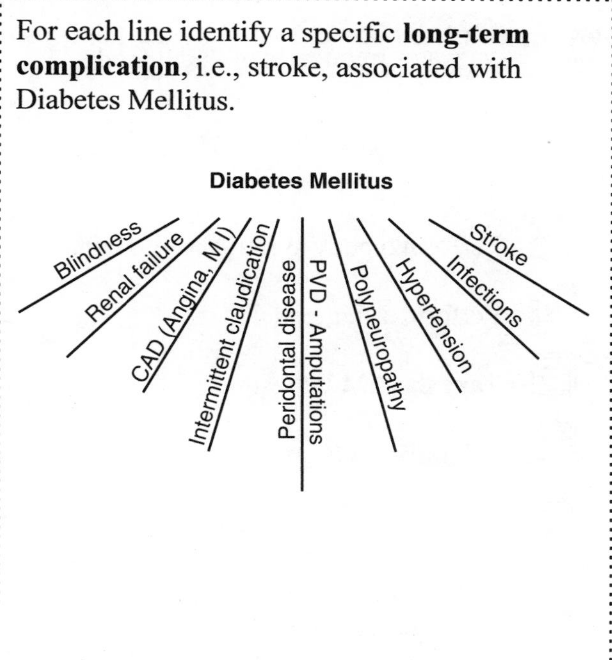

List the **causes** that precipitate the development of **Diabetic ketoacidosis**:

» Incorrect insulin dose or too little
» Omitting insulin dose
» Stress/Illness

Case Study: Mr. Edwards, 56 years old, has been a diabetic for 25 years. He has been in the hospital for a cerebral vascular accident for 3 days. His wife says that her husband monitors his blood sugars daily and administers his own insulin. However, she tells the nurse that he does not always stick to his diet. She wonders whether this may have contributed to the CVA. Mr. Edwards has an order for NPH insulin 36 U qAM and NPH 17 U qPM with blood sugar fingersticks ac and hs and he is started on a sliding scale.

Pertinent Terminology	Definition
Lipoatrophy	Characterized as a form of lipodystrophy. Atrophy of the SC fat developing depressions of the skin due to repeated injections.
Lipohypertrophy	Characterized as a form of lipodystrophy. The skin around the injection site overgrows resulting in bumpy or spongy appearance.
Impaired glucose tolerance	Blood sugar levels are higher than normal but not high enough to be classified as diabetes. A major risk factor for Type 2 DM.
Somogyi effect	Characterized by morning hyperglycemia with nocturnal or early morning hypoglycemia.
Dawn phenomenon	Noctural blood glucose normal until the early morning (3–4 AM) when there is rise of blood glucose.
Diabetic ketoacidosis	DKA—a state characterized by hyperglycemia, dehydration and excessive ketone bodies in the blood.
Hyperglycemic hyperosmolar nonketotic coma	(HHNK) A life-threatening condition, characterized by blood glucose >600 mg/dL, absence of acidosis and small to absent ketones.

Use the **case study, the follow-up information, and the nursing interventions below** to plan out Mr. Edward's morning care in the order of **priority**. Place a number, beginning with #1, in each box to indicate the sequence of the nursing care that should be delivered by the nurse.

Follow-up information: The AM blood sugar fingerstick and insulin are to be done by the morning shift. Mr. Edwards is started on a diet containing thick liquids.

	Nursing Interventions	Rationale
4	Perform a body systems assessment	Gather data.
1	Perform a fingerstick	Need to know AM fingerstick results
3	Take the AM vital signs	Gather data & establish baseline for the day.
2	Administer morning insulin	Maintain insulin levels. Correlate diet & insulin
5	Perform morning care	Assist patient, provide comfort.
7	Provide information regarding the complications of DM	Begin family/pt. teaching during hospital stay
6	Assist with breakfast	Ensure patient has adequate intake.

Place a check (✔) next to the statements that are correct regarding the use of a sliding scale.

_✔_ Only regular insulin is used

_✔_ Used for IDDM- Type 1 patients

_✔_ Dosage based on ac BS levels

_✔_ Used for NIDDM - Type 2 patients

_✔_ May be combined with other insulins

_✔_ Used during periods of illness

Interactive Activity: The following nursing diagnosis is found on Mr. Edwards' nursing care plan. With a partner, **write the 3 most important Nursing Interventions for the nursing diagnosis**.

Nursing Diagnosis	Nursing Interventions
Risk for Aspiration r/t impaired swallowing secondary to CVA	1. Sit in high Fowler's position for meals 2. Check for "pocketing" of food after each meal 3. Give thick liquids

THE PATIENT UNDERGOING SURGERY

(Development of signs and symptoms of shock)

Mr. Hatori, age 60, was admitted with persistent abdominal pain. He states he has had nausea and vomiting and has noticed a 10 lb weight loss within the last 2 months. He is diagnosed with gastric cancer and is scheduled for a subtotal gastrectomy in the morning. He has Demerol 75 mg with Phenergan 25 mg IM q3-4 hr prn pain and Mylanta 30 cc p.o. q2h prn abdominal pain. Mr. Hatori is very anxious after speaking with his physician and refuses to sign the surgical consent. He tells the nurse that he is having abdominal pain and "wants his pain shot right now." The nurse notes that it is just about three hours since his last pain medication.

Instructions: Prioritize the following **nursing interventions** as you, the nurse, would do them to initially take care of Mr. Hatori. Write a number in the box to identify the order of your interventions (#1 = first intervention, #2 = second intervention, etc.) and state a **rationale** for each intervention.

INTERVENTIONS	PRIORITY #	RATIONALE
◇ Administer IM pain med.	1	Pain management, provide comfort, decrease anxiety.
◇ Sit and talk with patient	3	Allay Mr. Hatori's anxiety. Assist in identifying concerns.
◇ Give Mylanta 30 cc	2	Pain management, provide comfort.
◇ Offer to call a family member	4	Solicit family support. Allay fears and anxiety.
◇ Notify physician	5	Inform physician of patient's concerns and assist patient to have his questions answered.

KEY POINTS TO CONSIDER:

Mr. Hatori does consent to have surgery and returns to the medical unit postoperative. He has an IV of lactated Ringer's infusing at 125 cc/hr and you note the following:

1) P. 90 - R. 20 - BP 130/76
2) He is alert, oriented, skin warm and dry
3) N/G tube draining brown-reddish drainage (300 cc in the last 4 hours)
4) Indwelling urinary catheter draining light yellow urine (700 cc in the last 4 hours)

✓✓✓ **Interactive Activity:** With a partner, **do the following: (1) based on the current assessment, select** the **one nursing diagnosis** that is priority at this time, **(2) provide a rationale** for your selection, and **(3) list three nursing interventions** that meet the needs of Mr. Hatori.

All of the following Nursing Diagnoses may apply to Mr. Hatori.

Risk for infection, Pain, Anxiety, Ineffective airway clearance, Fatigue, Impaired physical mobility, Altered nutrition: Less than body requirements, Knowledge deficit, Risk for fluid volume deficit, Fear.

Nursing Diagnosis	Rationale	Nursing Interventions
Risk for fluid volume deficit	Excessive loss of fluid also increases loss of Na^+ and hydrogen ions increasing risk of dehydration and electrolyte imbalance.	1. Maintain IV patency 2. Monitor I & O q1h 3. Monitor VS q2h

✓✓✓ Several hours after surgery you note that Mr. Hatori is very restless and you assess: R. 32 - P. 130 - BP 108/70, N/G drainage 200 cc bright red drainage, skin cool, c/o pain

Instructions: Based on the situation above, identify and write the **priority problem** in the box below. Then, starting with the small box labeled **#1, prioritize** the **nursing interventions** for this situation and **identify** your plan for follow-up care for Mr. Hatori.

NURSING INTERVENTIONS **DECISION-MAKING DIAGRAM**

A. Monitor P, R, BP
B. Document assessment/nursing care
C. Prepare for gastric lavage
D. Plan to start oxygen therapy
E. Stay with Mr. Hatori
F. Notify physician

Monitor VS 5-15 min.
Maintain IV therapy

New Action Plan

#1	#2	#3	#4	#5	#6
F	D	A	C	E	B

Signs and symptoms of shock

Priority Problem

NOTES

THE PATIENT WITH HEPATIC ENCEPHALOPATHY

(Development of signs and symptoms of impending coma)

Mr. Uribe, 47 yrs. old, is admitted with the diagnosis of hepatic encephalopathy related to his advanced cirrhosis of the liver. The night report indicates that he was awake most of the night and very restless most of shift. The nursing care kardex has the following orders:

VS q4hrs I & O (✔) Neuro cks q4hrs Serum ammonia, K^+ today Code Status: No code	D_5W at 100 cc/hr #20 g RFA - inserted today Bedrest with BRP Weigh daily	Diet: ↑ CHO, 50 g Prot., 4 g Na^+ Routine med: Neomycin 1 gm po q6h Lactulose 30 cc bid

As you enter his room you notice that Mr. Uribe is sleeping.

Instructions: Prioritize the five **nursing interventions** as you would do them to take care of Mr. Uribe. Write a number in the box to identify the order of your interventions (#1 = first intervention, #2 = second intervention, etc.) and state a **rationale** for each intervention.

INTERVENTIONS	PRIORITY #	RATIONALE
◇ Take the vital signs	2	Compare to previous recordings to detect changes
◇ Assess the LOC and orientation	1	Neurological changes may be subtle in the early stages.
◇ Check current serum ammonia and K^+ levels	4	Elevated serum ammonia levels are toxic to the CNS. Abnormal K^+ levels may cause cardiac irregularities.
◇ Perform a body systems physical assessment	3	Gather data.
◇ Assist Mr. Uribe with his ADLs	5	Activity & exercise increase the need glucose & protein as sources of energy. Protein breakdown increases ammonia.

KEY POINTS TO CONSIDER:

Mr. Uribe has refused his morning dose of lactulose and you further assess:

1) He refused the lactulose the previous day
2) No BM for 2 days
3) Irritable, speech slurred
4) Responds slowly to verbal communication

✓✓✓ **Interactive Activity:** With a partner, **do the following: (1) select** the **one nursing diagnosis** that is of priority at this time, **(2) provide a rationale** for your selection, and **(3) list the nursing interventions** that assist to meet the needs of the patient.

All of the following Nursing Diagnoses may apply to Mr. Uribe.

Risk for injury: Falls, Risk for infection, Impaired skin integrity, Self-care deficit: bathing/hygiene, Risk for impaired physical mobility, Risk for Constipation, Altered nutrition: Less than body requirements, Activity intolerance, Impaired tissue integrity, Fluid volume excess, Ineffective breathing pattern, Fatigue, Altered thought processes, Sleep pattern disturbance, Altered comfort.

Nursing Diagnosis	Rationale	Nursing Interventions
Risk for injury: Falls	Increased ammonia levels are toxic to the CNS affecting LOC, orientation, muscle twitching, etc.	1. Enc. fluid intake as ordered 2. Monitor VS & LOC 3. Bedrails ↑ at all times 4. Call light near patient

✓✓✓ You return from lunch at **1:00 p.m.** and you are informed of the following:

Mr. Uribe is becoming increasing confused and lethargic. He did not eat lunch.

Instructions: Based on the **1:00 p.m.** information, identify and write the **priority problem** in the box below. Then, starting with the small box labeled **#1, prioritize** the **nursing interventions** for this situation and **identify** your follow-up action plan for Mr. Uribe.

NURSING INTERVENTIONS

A. Inform RN/physician

B. Document assessment findings

C. Take the vital signs

D. Monitor neuro status

E. Stay with patient

F. Raise the bedrails

DECISION-MAKING DIAGRAM

Provide comfort & safety
Monitor VS & Neuro status
Notify relatives

New Action Plan

#1	#2	#3	#4	#5	#6
A	F	D	C	E	B

Signs and symptoms of impending coma

Priority Problem

NOTES______________________________

THE PATIENT UNDERGOING HEMODIALYSIS

(Development of signs and symptoms of disequilibrium syndrome)

Ms. Gladys Abbott, 52 yrs. old, has ESRD and has just been started on dialysis. She has an AV fistula in the right forearm and is scheduled for dialysis at 0800 today. The night nurse reports that the fistula has a good thrill and bruit. Ms. Abbott's BP is 160/102. You leave the report room at 0730 after noting the following orders from the nursing care kardex:

VS q8hrs I & O (✔) Weigh daily H & H, Serum Ferritin (✔) Serum Iron Saturation (✔)	IV: Saline lock - left hand Routine medications: Vasotec 10 mg po qd 0800 Folic acid 1 mg po qd 0800 $FeSo_4$ 325 po tid c̄ meals Epogen 300 U SC M-W-F	Diet: 70 g Protein, 2 g Na^+, 2 g K^+ Fluid restriction 1000 cc/day

Instructions: Prioritize the five **nursing interventions** as you would do them to take care of Ms. Abbott. Write a number in the box to identify the order of your interventions (#1 = first intervention, #2 = second intervention, etc.) and state a **rationale** for each intervention.

INTERVENTIONS	PRIORITY #	RATIONALE
◇ Take the VS (BP on the left arm)	2	Establish baseline. Avoid taking BP on right arm to prevent AV fistula from trauma.
◇ Perform body systems physical assessment	3	Establish baseline.
◇ Weigh patient/ensure Ms. Abbott has been weighed	4	Use as a guide to determine amount of fluid loss during dialysis treatment.
◇ Assess AV fistula for thrill & bruit	1	Assess patency of AV fistula.
◇ Hold folic acid and Vasotec	5	Water-soluble vitamins are lost during dialysis. Antihypertensives enhance hypotensive effects during treatment.

KEY POINTS TO CONSIDER:

Ordered lab studies were drawn prior to dialysis. The results of the morning lab are:

1) Hgb 9.5 g/dL, Hct 28%
2) Ferritin 60 ng/L
3) Serum iron saturation 18%
4) K^+ 5.0 mEq

✓✓✓ **Interactive Activity:** With a partner, **do the following: (1) select** the **one nursing diagnosis** that is of priority at this time, **(2) provide a rationale** for your selection, and **(3) list the nursing interventions** that assist to meet the needs of the patient.

All of the following Nursing Diagnoses may apply to Ms. Abbott.

Risk for injury, Knowledge deficit, Fear, Anxiety, Risk for infection, Impaired tissue integrity, Risk for Alteration in sensory/perceptual, Constipation, Fluid volume excess, Fluid volume deficit, Body image disturbance, Risk for impaired physical mobility, Altered tissue perfusion, Altered nutrition: Less than body requirements, Fatigue.

Nursing Diagnosis	Rationale	Nursing Interventions
Fatigue	Anemia causes a reduction in the oxygen carrying capacity of the blood leading to tissue hypoxia.	1. Plan periods of rest after activities 2. Enc. adequate intake 3. Nutritional consult to inc. iron-rich foods in diet 4. Monitor H & H

✓✓✓ **After the dialysis treatment,** Ms. Abbott is restless and you assess:

c/o headache, pruritis, nausea, change in LOC, twitching, confusion

Instructions: Based on **after the dialysis treatment** data, identify and write the **priority problem** in the box below. Then, starting with the small box labeled **#1, prioritize** the **nursing interventions** for this situation and **identify** your follow-up action plan for Ms. Abbott.

NURSING INTERVENTIONS

A. Take the VS

B. Notify RN/physician

C. Maintain calm, quiet environment

D. Stay with patient

E. Monitor neuro status

F. Document assessment findings

DECISION-MAKING DIAGRAM

Monitor vital signs and neuro status
Seizure precautions

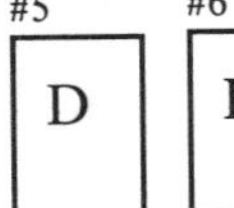

New Action Plan

#1	#2	#3	#4	#5	#6
A	B	E	C	D	F

Signs and symptoms of disequilibrium syndrome

Priority Problem

NOTES__________

THE PATIENT WITH UROSEPSIS

(Development of signs and symptoms of septic shock)

Mr. Tyler, 79 yrs. old, was admitted today to the hospital with the Dx. of Urosepsis. He has an IV of D_5/0.45 NS infusing at 100 cc/hr. Rocephin 1 gm IVPB qd is ordered. He is on I & O q8hr, soft diet, BRP with assistance and Tylenol tabs ii p.o. q4h for temp >38. The day shift nurse indicated his VS were T. 38°C - P. 78 - R. 22 BP 146/88 at 2:00 PM. The nurse also said that he was more restless this afternoon and had been trying to get out of bed and seemed somewhat disoriented. He did not receive Tylenol but an order for a vest restraint was obtained and has been applied. You have been assigned as his nurse for the evening shift.

Instructions: Prioritize the following **nursing interventions** as you, the nurse, would do them to initially take care of Mr. Tyler. Write a number in the box to identify the order of your interventions (#1 = first intervention, #2 = second intervention, etc.) and state a **rationale** for each intervention.

INTERVENTIONS	PRIORITY #	RATIONALE
◇ Administer Tylenol tabs ii p.o. if necessary	2	Monitor changes in temperature.
◇ Take the vital signs	1	Reassess VS—especially temp.
◇ Gather urinary output data	4	Assess amount and voiding pattern.
◇ Check the vest restraint	5	Safety precautions. Prevent patient injury.
◇ Perform a body systems physical assessment	3	Establish baseline. Assess bladder. May have a full bladder and this may contribute to his restlessness.

KEY POINTS TO CONSIDER:

You perform a follow-up assessment at 7:00 PM and note the following:

1) VS - T. 38.5°C - P. 88 - R. 22 BP 120/76
2) Fine crackles audible on auscultation in the bilateral lower lung fields
3) He is sleepy.
4) He was incontinent of a scant amount of urine.

✓✓✓ **Interactive Activity:** With a partner, **do the following: (1) select** the **one nursing diagnosis** that is of priority at this time, **(2) provide a rationale** for your selection, and **(3) list the nursing interventions** that assist to meet the needs of the patient:

All of the following Nursing Diagnoses may apply to Mr. Tyler.

Risk for impaired skin integrity, Altered urinary elimination, Risk for injury, Altered thought processes, Hyperthermia, Fluid volume deficit, Altered nutrition: Less than body requirements, Ineffective breathing pattern, Fatigue.

Nursing Diagnosis	Rationale	Nursing Interventions
Hyperthermia	Infectious processes alter the temperature control center in the hypothalmus by increasing the thermo-regulatory mechanisms in the brain.	1. Administer Tylenol 2. Maintain IV patency 3. Enc. fluids q2h 4. C & DB q1h 5. Monitor vital signs

✓✓✓As you take his **8:00 PM** VS you note the following signs and symptoms on Mr. Tyler:

Lethargic, skin very warm and flushed, VS - T. 39.1°C - P. 130 - R. 28 BP 90/54

Instructions: Based on the **8:00 PM** situation above, identify and write the **priority problem** in the box below. Then, starting with the small box labeled **#1, prioritize** the **nursing interventions** for this situation and **identify** your follow-up action plan for Mr. Tyler.

NURSING INTERVENTIONS

A. Check oxygen saturation level
B. Place in modified Trendelenburg position
C. Prepare to insert indwelling urinary catheter
D. Take vital signs
E. Document findings
F. Notify RN/physician

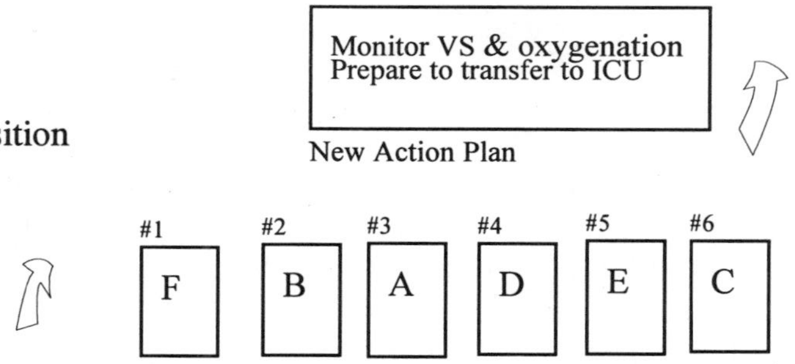

DECISION-MAKING DIAGRAM

New Action Plan: Monitor VS & oxygenation
Prepare to transfer to ICU

#1	#2	#3	#4	#5	#6
F	B	A	D	E	C

Priority Problem: Signs & symptoms of septic shock

NOTES____________________

THE PATIENT WITH A FRACTURED TIBIA

(Development of signs and symptoms of compartment syndrome)

Mr. F. Williams, 26 yrs. old, was admitted with a left fractured tibia. He was taken to surgery and is now being transferred to the Orthopedic Unit. He has a long leg cast on the left leg. His postop orders are transcribed to the nursing care kardex:

VS q4hrs I & O (✔) Neurovascular cks (circ. movement, sensation, temp) q4hr Elevate left leg on (1) pillow	1L D_5W q10hrs—dc when taking fluids well Teach crutch walking in AM	Diet: Clear liquids → Reg. PRN med: Meperidine 100 mg IM q4h prn pain

You are assigned to Mr. Williams as he is taken into his room. You note that he is alert, left leg cast is damp and clean, IV is infusing into right hand.

Instructions: Prioritize the five **nursing interventions** as you would do them to take care of Mr. Williams. Write a number in the box to identify the order of your interventions (#1 = first intervention, #2 = second intervention, etc.) and state a **rationale** for each intervention.

INTERVENTIONS	PRIORITY #	RATIONALE
◇ Take the vital signs	1	Establish baseline. Compare to the previous recordings.
◇ Neurovascular assessment of both extremities	2	Establish baseline. Compare circulation, movement, sensation and pedal pulses.
◇ Assess cast for dryness, signs of drainage, and sharp edges	4	Establish baseline, gather data, and assess for areas of increased heat, drainage and odor.
◇ Use palms of hands to elevate cast on a pillow	3	Safety. Prevent indentations to cast and promote circulation.
◇ Teach isometric exercises	5	Assist to maintain muscle mass and strength.

KEY POINTS TO CONSIDER:

On the morning of the first postop day, you note that Mr. Williams is:

1) Requesting pain med q4hrs
2) Left pedal pulses present, edema 2+
3) Capillary refill >2 sec, moves left toes
4) Taking fluids and voiding qs
5) M.D. orders CPK, LDH, and SGOT

✓✓✓ **Interactive Activity:** With a partner, **do the following: (1) select** the **one nursing diagnosis** that is of priority at this time, **(2) provide a rationale** for your selection, and **(3) list the nursing interventions** that assist to meet the needs of the patient.

All of the following Nursing Diagnoses may apply to Mr. Williams.

Risk for injury, Knowledge deficit, Risk for infection, Risk for impaired skin integrity, Risk for impaired physical mobility, Fear, Altered tissue perfusion: peripheral, Pain, Activity intolerance, Impaired tissue integrity, Anxiety, Risk for peripheral neurovascular dysfunction.

Nursing Diagnosis	Rationale	Nursing Interventions
Risk for peripheral neurovascular dysfunction	Presence of edema increases the risk of tissue pressure and decreases blood supply.	1. Ensure extremity is elevated 2. Neurovascular checks q1h 3. Monitor for c/o inc. pain

✓✓✓ **Mr. Williams refuses lunch** and you assess:

c/o increased pain, esp. with elevation of leg, numbness & tingling, left pedal pulse weak, cool

Instructions: Based on the fact that **Mr. Williams refuses lunch**, identify and write the **priority problem** in the box below. Then, starting with the small box labeled **#1, prioritize** the **nursing interventions** for this situation and **identify** your follow-up action plan for Mr. Williams.

NURSING INTERVENTIONS

A. Inform RN/MD stat
B. Prepare to have cast bivalved
C. Ensure left extremity is at heart level
D. Monitor left pedal pulse
E. Take the vital signs
F. Stay with patient

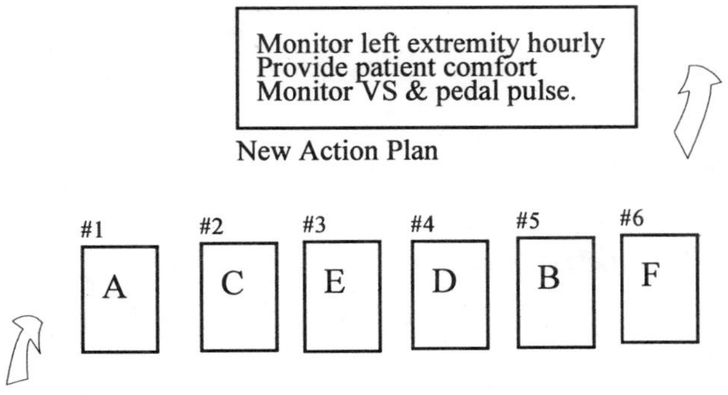

DECISION-MAKING DIAGRAM

Monitor left extremity hourly
Provide patient comfort
Monitor VS & pedal pulse.

New Action Plan

#1	#2	#3	#4	#5	#6
A	C	E	D	B	F

Signs and symptoms of compartment syndrome

Priority Problem

NOTES____________________

THE PATIENT WITH CATARACT SURGERY

(Development of signs and symptoms of intraocular pressure)

Mrs. Tami Fields, 72 yrs. old, has senile cataracts and has been instilling mydriatic eye gtts. Her vision has progressively worsened and is scheduled today for a right cataract extraction in the outpatient clinic. The M.D. orders the following preop preparation: NPO, instill myriatic and cycloplegic eye gtts 1 hour prior to surgery, Valium 5 mg po 1 hour prior to surgery. Mrs. Fields arrives at the outpatient clinic at 0800 and she is scheduled for surgery at 1000.

Instructions: Prioritize the five **nursing interventions** as you would do them to take care of Mrs. Fields. Write a number in the box to identify the order of your interventions (#1 = first intervention, #2 = second intervention, etc.) and state a **rationale** for each intervention.

INTERVENTIONS	PRIORITY #	RATIONALE
◇ Provide information regarding preop preparation	2	Providing information ↓ pt. anxiety and ↑ pt. cooperation.
◇ Begin to instill ordered eye gtts	4	Begin preop preparation as ordered to dilate eye prior to surgery.
◇ Have patient void	5	Preop preparation and decrease patient discomfort during surgical procedure.
◇ Take the vital signs	3	Establish baseline to compare subsequent vital signs.
◇ Ensure the surgical consent	1	Ensure consent is signed prior to initiating preop preparation to address pt. concerns and legal considerations.

KEY POINTS TO CONSIDER:

Mrs. Fields had an intraocular lens implant and is taken to the recovery room. She has an eye patch on her right eye and you assess the following:

1) No c/o pain, P. 88, BP 130/82
2) Eye patch clean and dry
3) Readily responds to verbal stimuli

✓✓✓ **Interactive Activity:** With a partner, **do the following: (1) select** the **one nursing diagnosis** that is of priority at this time, **(2) provide a rationale** for your selection, and **(3) list the nursing interventions** that assist to meet the needs of the patient:

All of the following Nursing Diagnoses may apply to Mrs. Fields.

Risk for injury, Knowledge deficit, Sensory-perceptual alterations: visual, Fear, Anxiety, Risk for self-care deficit, Risk for infection, Altered health maintenance, Impaired home maintenance management.

Nursing Diagnosis	Rationale	Nursing Interventions
Sensory-perceptual alterations: visual	Patch eye will decrease visual fields and visual perceptions	1. Orient to environment 2. Educate pt./family re: environmental safety, eye care 3. Ensure adequate lighting

✓✓✓ One hour **postop** you assess Mrs. Fields and note the following:

c/o right brow pain, anxious, P. 110, BP 128/80 coughing and c/o nausea

Instructions: Based on the **postop** assessment, identify and write the **priority problem** in the box below. Then, starting with the small box labeled **#1, prioritize** the **nursing interventions** for this situation and **identify** your follow-up action plan for Mrs. Fields.

NURSING INTERVENTIONS

A. Avoid rapid head movement

B. Administered antiemetic if ordered

C. Document findings/nursing care

D. Notify M.D.

E. Recheck pulse and BP

F. Stay with Mrs. Fields

DECISION-MAKING DIAGRAM

Monitor VS and pain level Avoid pressure on operative side. Reassure patient.

New Action Plan

#1	#2	#3	#4	#5	#6
D	B	A	E	F	C

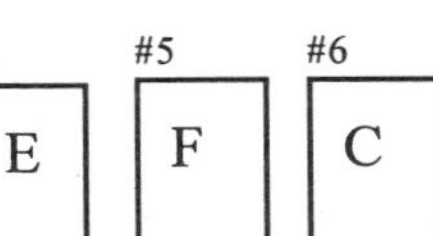

Signs and symptoms of intraocular pressure

Priority Problem

NOTES

CLINICAL SITUATION - # 1
(Small bowel resection with postop care)

Intershift taped report at 0700:

"Mr. Andrews, 72 yrs. old, is 2 days postop small bowel resection. His N/G tube is connected to low wall suction and is draining dark brown fluid. Vital signs at 0600: T. 99.6° - P. 90 – R. 28 160/94. IV D_5/0.45 NS with 20 mEq KCl infusing at 125 cc into the right forearm. He is using the PCA machine. He slept most of the night and is now sitting in a chair. SOB was noted when he was transferred to the chair. There are 300 cc left in the IV."

Mr. Andrews' current **flow charts** contain the following information:

Medication Record

Routine	Time Due
Lanoxin 0.25 mg IV qd	0900
Lasix 20 mg IVP qd	0900
Timolol 0.25% gtt ⫟ OU bid	1000
Zantac 50 mg IVPB q6h	1000
Gentamicin 80 mg IVPB q8h	1400

PRN
Phenergan 25 mg IV/IM q4h prn/V
PCA (morphine sulfate – 1 mg/hr)

Intake and Output Record

Night Shift @ 0600

Intake		Output	
P.O.	= 0	UA void	= 0
		Foley	= 200
IV	= 1000	N/G	= 600
IVPB	= 100		

Interactive activity: With a partner, **use the case study and the flow charts** to:

1. Identify the pertinent patient information made known to you in the report	2. Identify the pertinent information you gathered from the flow charts	3. Review the data in columns 1 & 2 and identify information that needs follow-up
● 2-days postop bowel resection.	● Has Lanoxin and Lasix ordered	◆ GI assessment: Bowel sounds/NG tube Abd dressing/incision
● Has N/G to low wall suction; draining dark brown fluid.	● Timolol gtts indicates treatment for glaucoma	◆ Collect data previous VS recordings. Reassess VS
● Has IV in the RFA with 300 cc left and is using the PCA.	● Morphine is used in the PCA	◆ Perform physical exam focus on CV, Resp., Skin
● Vital signs out of the normal range.	● Foley output 200 cc for the night shift	◆ Gather data as to IV insertion date
● Currently experienced SOB	● N/G output 600 cc	◆ Assess current lab, especially electrolytes

It is 0730 as you leave the report room, **prioritize** your plan of care for the morning:

Time	Plan of Nursing Care
0730	Get further report from RN. Check medications.
0745	Perform body systems assessment. Check N/G tube and Foley output. Assess IV and IV fluid. Reassess VS. Get next IV bag ready.
0815	Document assessment findings. Check results of current lab work.
0845	Prepare IV medications. Hang up new IV bag. Enc. C & DB
0900	Take apical pulse, administer IV medications.
0915	Provide or ensure that care is given.
1000	Assess IV/PCA. Monitor resp. and output. Administer eye gtts. IVPB
1100	Document any additional findings. Maintain comfort.

1200 nursing assessment: Oriented x3, skin WNL, capillary refill < 3 sec., turgor good, mucous membranes moist, pinkish, T. 99, P. 88 slightly irregular, R. 24, BP 164/94. N/G draining brownish fluid 100 cc since 0800. Bowel sounds present x4, abd. soft. Foley catheter draining clear yellow urine.

Mr. Andrews has minimal complaints and is visited by the physician at 1200. The physician leaves the following orders:

Remove Foley now
Enc. incentive spirometer q1h x10
Discontinue N/G tube
DC Lasix
Lanoxin 0.25 mg po qd
Hgb & Hct today
Clear liquid diet

1. Identify the nursing interventions that require immediate follow-up	**2. Identify the nursing actions that you can delegate/assign to unlicensed personnel**
Remove Foley Discontinue N/G tube Discuss with physician the BP, esp. since Lasix was discontinued	Enc. incentive spirometer q1h x10 Make sure Mr. Andrews gets his tray Maintain I & O

For each of the following **nursing interventions**, write an **expected patient outcome**:

1. Foley removed at 1300 ⇨ Will void within 6 - 8 hours.

2. Incentive spirometer q1h x10 ⇨ Lungs will remain clear throughout hosp. stay

CLINICAL SITUATION - # 5
(Patient with pancreatitis and central line)

Intershift taped report at 3:00 PM:

"Mrs. Clark, 42 yrs. old, was admitted earlier today with acute pancreatitis. She had midepigastric pain with nausea and vomiting on admission. Her latest vitals signs are T. 38°C - P. 108 - R. 26 BP 110/60. Bowel sounds are hypoactive. I medicated her at 2:00 PM. A central line was inserted, you have 800 cc left in the IV. The N/G is draining brownish fluid. She needs to have the urinary catheter inserted."

Mrs. Clark's current **flow charts** contain the following information:

Patient Care Kardex

VS: q4hrs Diet: NPO
O2 @ 3L/NP
Pulse oximetry q4hrs

IV: D_5W @125 cc/hr
Right central line
N/G tube to low con't suction ☑
Urinary catheter inserted ☐

ABG in AM ☐
K^+, Na^+, Cl^-, CO_2, Mg^{2+}, Ca^{++} in AM ☐
Abd CT scan @ 6 PM today

Routine Medication:
Cimetidine 300 mg IVPB q6h 10-4-10-4

PRN Medication:
Meperidine 75 mg IM q3h prn pain

Admission Lab Data

Se Amylase 350 units/L
Se Lipase 260 units/L

Hgb 11.6 g/dL
Hct 32%
WBC 18,000/mm^3

LDH 300 units/L
AST 80 units/L

BS 200 mg/dL

Interactive activity: With a partner, **use the case study and the flow charts** to:

1. Identify the pertinent patient information made known to you in the report	2. Identify the pertinent information you gathered from the flow charts	3. Review the data in columns 1 & 2 and identify information that needs follow-up
● Admitted earlier today	● O_2 @ 3L/NP pulse oximetry	◆ Assess IV, central line, N/G tube, drainage
● Midepigastric pain with nausea & vomiting	● Cimetidine IVPB @ 4 PM and 10 PM	◆ Perform a body systems assessment
● 38 - 108 - 26 110/60	● IV at 125 cc/hr	◆ Check oxygen settings/ pulse oximetry
● Bowel sounds hypoactive	● VS q 4hr	◆ Insert urinary catheter
● IV and central line	● Abd CT scan today	◆ Assess pain level
● N/G tube to low suction	● All lab data abnormal	◆ Monitor for complications

It is 4:00 PM, prioritize your plan of care for the next three hours:

Time	Plan of Nursing Care
4:00 PM	Assess central line, IV fluid, hang up IVPB. Assess pain level. Perform a body systems assessment, take vital signs, check pulse oximetry, N/G tube and drainage.
4:30	Insert urinary catheter.
5:30	Document findings. Prepare for CT scan. Assess pain level.
6:00	To CT scan.
	Reassess patient, IV, central line, N/G, oxygen level, urinary catheter, upon return from CT scan.

At 8:30 PM the nursing assistant informs you that Mrs. Clark is complaining of pain and is restless. You note that she has not had a pain shot in the last three hours. You walk into the room to assess her and to give her a meperidine injection. She turns over quickly and pulls out the central line.

1. Identify the nursing interventions that you would implement immediately at the bedside	**2. Identify the follow-up nursing actions. Document the incident in the nurse's notes.**
Cover central line site and apply pressure	Call physician
Assess respiratory status, pulse rate	Monitor pulse oximetry
Monitor for complaints of chest pain	

Nurse's Notes

8:30 PM c/o pain, turned in bed, central line pulled out completely. Pressure applied over site for 5 minutes. Vital signs taken. Respirations unlabored. Denies chest pain. Physician notified.

For the following **nursing intervention**, write the **expected patient outcome**:

1. Call physician regarding abnormal lab values 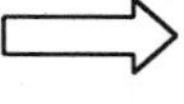 Blood sugar will be WNL after implementation of physician order (insulin administration).

CLINICAL SITUATION - # 10
(Elderly patient with MRSA)

Intershift taped report at 11:00 PM:

"Mrs. Jaffey, 88 yrs. old, was admitted this evening from a nursing home after the family found her lethargic and confused. Her admitting vital signs were T 101°F - P. 92 - irregular - R. 28 short and shallow and BP 110/70. Her physician was called for admitting orders, he will come in tomorrow morning to see her. She was given Tylenol at 8:30 PM and her current temp. is 100.6, she is still slightly confused. The family states that she had cataract surgery one week ago as an outpatient. She has an IV going. The patient in the next bed is concerned about Mrs. Jaffey's moaning."

Mrs. Jaffey's current **flow charts** contain the following information:

Nursing Care Kardex

VS q4h Diet: DAT

LBM: On admission
IV: 0.9% NS at 75 cc/hr
#24 angio cath RFA

Lab: CBC, Chem panel, UA

PRN Medication:
Tylenol 325 mg tabs ii q4hrs prn temp > 101

Nurse's Notes from Skilled Nursing Facility

Documentation of latest nurse's notes:

1600 Turned, incontinent of urine, strong urine odor, incontinent pad applied. *A. Cann LVN*
1700 Family in to visit. Upset, called physician. *A. Cann LVN*
1830 Transferred to hospital per order. Recent UA culture reports show + MRSA. Unable to contact physician, copy of report included with transfer. *T. Gage RN*

Interactive activity: With a partner, **use the case study and the flow charts** to:

1. Identify the pertinent patient information made known to you in the report	2. Identify the pertinent information you gathered from the flow charts	3. Review the data in columns 1 & 2 and identify information that needs follow-up
• Admitted from a nursing • Lethargic and confused • Had temp; received Tylenol • Had cataract surgery one week ago • Current temp. 100.6°F • She is in a room with another patient	• Incontinent of urine • Family upset • UA culture + MRSA • Physician not aware of	◆ Perform a body systems assessment ◆ Inform physician of MRSA report ◆ Transfer Mrs. Jaffey to isolation/private room ◆ Reassess vital signs

It is 11:30 PM, prioritize your plan of care for the next hour:

Time	Plan of Nursing Care
11:30 PM	Take vital signs, perform assessment, place call to physician, check for room availability.
12:00 AM	Document findings.
12:30 AM	Follow hospital policy for care of MRSA patients (isolation, equipment, etc.).

Mrs. Jaffey is moved to a private room with isolation set up. She slept 1 - 2 hours at a time during the night and remains confused. She has developed a productive cough and is expectorating a small amount of thick creamy yellow-colored phlegm. Her morning vital signs are, T. 100.8°F - P. 110 - R. 32 - BP 114/82. At 6:30 AM the physician visits and leaves the following orders:

Vancomycin 500 mg q6h IVPB
Insert indwelling urinary catheter
Bedrest
Chest x-ray/ECG
Oxygen 2 L/min/NP, pulse oximeter q4hrs
I & O, enc. fluid intake

1. Identify the nursing interventions that you would plan to implement immediately	**2. Identify the instructions you would give to staff and family in caring for Mrs. Jaffey**
Start oxygen 2 L/min/NP	Washing hands frequently
Monitor oxygen saturation	Offer fluids frequently
Insert indwelling urinary catheter	Turn q2hrs
Order chest x-ray and ECG	Cough and deep breathe q1h while awake

For the following **nursing intervention**, write an **expected patient outcome**:

1. Encourage fluid intake 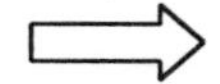 Will have ↓ thickness of sputum; maintain patent airway

CLINICAL SITUATION - # 15
(Patient with hip fracture and DVT)

Intershift taped report at 7:00 AM:

"Mrs. LaVerne, 74 yrs. old, is four days postop left hip fracture. She had a constavac that was removed yesterday. Surgical dressing is clean and dry. Pedal pulse on the left foot is present and the circulation, movement and sensation are WNL. Lung sounds with fine crackles at the lower bases in both lungs. You need to encourage her to deep breaths and use the incentive spirometer. Her 6:00 AM vital signs are T. 99.8°F - P. 80 - R. 18 BP 130/82. She does not want to move, it seems like she is scared. I have medicated her two times during the night."

Mrs. LaVerne's current **flow charts** contain the following information:

Nursing Care Kardex

VS: qs   Diet: Soft
HOH   I & O
Ambulate with PT

LBM (2 days ago)

IV: Saline lock LFA #22 g angio cath
Inserted day of surgery

Routine Medications:

Digoxin 0.125 mg po qd	9
Furosemide 10 mg po qd	9
$FeSO_4$ 300 mg po TID c̄ meals	8-12-5

PRN:
Vicodin tab ⫱ q4h prn pain

Medical History

Elderly female brought into the ED after falling at home. A fracture of the Left hip was diagnosed. She was taken to surgery and an ORIF was performed. Hgb 9.4 mg/dL, Hct 28% on admission.

She lives alone, has one son and her husband died two years ago from a cardiac condition.

Patient has a history of atrial fibrillation.

Interactive activity: With a partner, **use the case study and the flow charts** to:

1. Identify the pertinent patient information made known to you in the <u>report</u>	2. Identify the pertinent information you gathered from the <u>flow charts</u>	3. Review the data in columns 1 & 2 and identify information that needs follow-up
• 74 years old • Pedal pulse present L foot Circulation, movement & sensation WNL • Lungs sounds with fine crackles • 99.8 - 80 - 18 130/82 • Scared does not want to move • Dressing is clean and dry • Medicated 2x during the night	• HOH • Ambulate with PT • Saline lock LFA -inserted since surgery • Hgb 9.4 mg/dL, Hct 28% • History of atrial fibrillation • 8 & 9 AM medications • Lives alone • LBM two days ago	◆ Assess respiratory status ◆ Assess pedal pulses ◆ Perform a body systems assessment ◆ Plan to change IV site ◆ Assess dressing and (L) leg ◆ Assess pulse rhythm

It is 7:30 AM, prioritize your plan of care for the next hour:

Time	Plan of Nursing Care
7:30 AM	Assess left leg and surgical dressing. Perform a full body systems assessment.
	Assess respiratory status and IV site.
	Prepare for breakfast. Prepare to administer 8:00 AM medication

 **You review the nurse's notes from the night shift and note the following:**

12:00 PM Alert, moaning, states leg hurts. Circulation, movement, and sensation of left leg WNL. Dressing clean and dry. Repositioned. Vicodin tab† given for pain.
2:00 AM Awake, states pain in leg, does not want to be touched. Left pedal pulse palpable. Repositioned.
4:00 AM Sleeping
6:00 AM c/o leg pain . Medicated with Vicodin tab†.

You enter the following assessment in the nurse's notes:
7:30 AM Awake, alert, states "did not have a good night." c/o leg pain. Left leg with pedal pulse, warm, cap. refill >2 secs. Leg elevated on pillow. Dressing clean and dry. Right leg with weak pedal pulse, swelling and redness noted at calf and thigh. Tender to touch. Lung sounds with fine crackles, encouraged to take deep breaths. Bowel sounds present x4, c/o constipation.

1. Identify the nursing interventions that require immediate follow-up.	**2. Identify the instructions that you will give the nursing assistants at this time.**
Maintain bedrest Call physician Elevate right leg	Maintain bedrest Avoid use of knee gatch Do not massage right leg Vital signs q4h Notify nurse stat if patient experiences SOB or chest pain Maintain right leg elevated

For the following **nursing intervention**, write the **expected patient outcome**:

1. Elevation of right leg 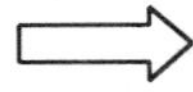 Swelling will decrease; venous return will be enhanced.

CLINICAL SITUATION - # 20
(Patient with TAH and epidural catheter)

Intershift taped report at 7:00 AM:

"Mrs. Farrell, 46 yrs. old, had a TAH-BSO yesterday. She had soft bowel sounds this morning. The abdominal dressing is clean and dry. Her IV is infusing well and she has an epidural infusion with fentanyl infusing through a pump. She has not had any breakthrough pain. The epidural dressing is intact and the catheter is fine. She has been mostly on bedrest, but she is to get up to a chair this morning. The 6:00 AM vital signs are T. 37.5°C - P. 78 - R. 18 130/80. Her output was 500 cc."

Mrs. Farrell's current **flow charts** contain the following information:

Nursing Care Rand

VS: q4s Diet: Clear liquids
Up in chair with assistance
Incentive spirometer q1h x10 WA
LBM: Prior to admission

Urinary catheter ☑

IV: D5/0.45 NS q8hrs

Routine Medication:
Fentanyl 6 cc/hr in NS via epidural catheter ordered by anesthesiologist

Intake and Output Record

Night shift:

Intake		Output	
Oral: (Sips of H_2O)	50	Void	
		UA cath	500
IV:	1000		
IV	48		

Interactive activity: With a partner, **use the case study and the flow charts** to:

1. Identify the pertinent patient information made known to you in the report	2. Identify the pertinent information you gathered from the flow charts	3. Review the data in columns 1 & 2 and identify information that needs follow-up
• TAH-BSO yesterday • Soft bowel sounds • Abd. dressing is clean & dry • IV is infusing well • Has epidural infusion with fentanyl • No breakthrough pain • 37.5 - 78 - 18 130/80	• VS q4hrs • Clear liquid diet • IV q8hrs • Urinary catheter • Inc. spirometer q1h x10	◆ Assess epidural infusion and catheter ◆ Perform a body systems assessment ◆ Assess IV ◆ Have patient use incentive spirometer ◆ Assess urinary catheter and output

It is 7:30 AM, prioritize your plan of care for the next hour:

Time	Plan of Nursing Care
7:30 AM	Assess epidural catheter and site, pump, fentanyl bottle, and pain control.
	Assess IV and IV site. Perform a body systems assessment. Assess vital signs.
	Assess surgical dressing. Assess urinary catheter, output.
	Document findings.

At 8:30 AM Mrs. Farrell gets up with assistance to sit in a chair. As she walks slowly to the chair, she steps on some of the tubings. The nursing assistance tells you that the infusion pump is beeping. You go into assess and note that the epidural infusion pump is beeping and the patient's epidural dressing is pulled from the patient's back. The epidural catheter seems to be pulled out.

1. Identify the nursing interventions that you would plan to implement immediately	**2. Document your findings as you would enter them in a nursing notes.**
Cover epidural site with a 4x4 Put patient back to bed Notify the anesthesiologist Turn off the pump Monitor pulse, resp. BP	**Nursing Notes** 8:30 AM. Up to chair with assistance. Epidural infusion tubing accidentally pulled out upon transfer to chair. Anesthesiologist notified. VS taken. Patient assisted back to bed.

For each of the following **nursing intervention**, write an **expected patient outcome**:

1. Cover epidural site with 4x4 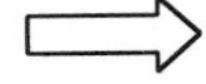 Will minimize bacterial invasion; will provide protection to epidural site.